Tapping and Eft

Quick and Simple Exercises to De-stress

(A Beginner's Simple Step Plan to Overcome Emotional Problems)

Dennis Woodyard

Published By **Elena Holly**

Dennis Woodyard

Tapping and Eft: Quick and Simple Exercises to De-stress (A Beginner's Simple Step Plan to Overcome Emotional Problems)

ISBN 978-1-7770981-3-1

Legal & Disclaimer

Table Of Contents

Chapter 1: Eft Tapping

What is EFT?

EFT stands for Emotional Freedom Technique.

It could be compared to Emotional Acupuncture, but without needles. It's also been described as a type of acupressure that is combined with concentration on the mind. It's actually a basic technique for stress-reduction that is based on the traditional Chinese energetic meridian method, the same system of meridian that's been utilized for the past five thousand years or for Acupuncture. The practice of using it for SO many years tells me that it's effective otherwise they'd have dropped the practice long ago.

EFT utilizes the similar "energy meridian system" that is employed in Acupuncture however instead of needles you apply pressure to certain energy meridian points in the body using your fingers. While Acupuncture is typically focused on physical issues, EFT is usually focused on the emotional aspect of things. However, the great thing with EFT is that, often through "clearing" the "stuck energy" that is associated with the emotional side that the physical aspect will also get better. A lot of people utilize EFT to tackle physical problems by focusing on their thoughts, thoughts and emotions that are associated with the physical problem.

Disclaimer

Before we start before we begin, I must give you this disclaimer (in addition to the one I provided that was in my book earlier!):

And I'm not a doctor and I'm not even one on television.

The information provided here is intended for only informational purposes.

+ The techniques, ideas and suggestions that are presented herein are not intended to be an alternative to consulting with a licensed health professional.

Many people have seen great results with EFT however, it's still seen as an experimental method.

If you have questions about whether or how to make use of EFT you should consult your doctor or licensed health specialist.

+ Do not stop any treatment or medication without the supervision of a doctor.

And you must accept the responsibility for your actions I am not responsible for, or be held accountable for, your actions and decisions. Only you can make that decision.

+ EFT is trademark registered of the company's creator Gary Craig.

+ Gary is now been laid off as well as "Given EFT to the world" however Gary is not associated or influence over the information presented here.

It's my interpretation of EFT that is based upon all of my training, from Gary Craig and others.

Origins of EFT

Gary Craig, a Stanford University trained engineer, developed EFT around 1993, in the year 1993 based on the concepts that he was taught by the late Dr. Roger Callahan, a classically trained clinical psychologist. The doctor. Callahan who made the first discoveries that established the foundation for the current tapping techniques are built.

Doctor. Callahan was working with one of his patients named Mary. She was plagued by an INTENSE fear of water from the time she was a child. The fear of water was so intense for her that she could not even bathe in a tub filled with water! She even feared each rainy day and she would have nightmares concerning "water getting her."

Doctor. Callahan had been using traditional psychotherapy methods with her for nearly nothing happening. The most they were accomplished was having Mary hang her legs over the water at the edge of the pool and not gaze towards the pool. After each session, she was left with severe headaches due to the tension.

In dismay at their lack of improvement and lack of progress, Dr. Callahan was looking outside of the conventional methods and was studying Energie Meridians from Acupuncture. Mary frequently mentioned that drinking water caused her to feel an unpleasant sensation in her stomach. The doctor. Callahan decided to try an experiment, and demanded Mary to tap the side of stomach meridian that is located directly beneath the eyes.

In his amazement, Mary said, "It's gone! The numb feeling I feel in my stomach whenever I think of the water is disappeared!" At first, the doctor was skeptical but she immediately leapt up and ran towards the pool without hesitation. Doctor. Callahan was concerned because she was unable to swim, however Mary assured him that, no matter how much fear was gone, because she was aware that she wasn't able to swim, it didn't mean she was stupid.

After that the doctor. Callahan went on to create the technique in a more advanced manner and, after a series of other research and experiments with other patients, he created Thought Field Therapy, or TFT. The technique he developed included a few diagnostic steps and different tapping "recipes," that differed according to what the issue was for the patient. He devised a number different recipes which he has used effectively with a range of patients and ailments. He has been able to help many patients with various fears, fears and life-related traumas, too.

Then, a few years later, Gary Craig took some instruction with the Dr. Callahan on the tapping method he invented. With the eyes of an Stanford University trained engineer, Gary realized the possibility of simplifying and broaden the TFT technique, including its complicated diagnostic steps and tap "recipes", into a more simple type of tapping that is now referred to as EFT also known as Emotional Freedom Technique.

There are many variants and modifications that are related to EFT They all fall under the general name of Tapping Modalities. Whatever their variations might have, they operate by tapping the body's energy Meridian system.

What is the process behind EFT function?

Although there are a myriad various theories proposed as to the way EFT operates, nobody can be sure. Gary came to a plausible explanation in the EFT Thesis statement, which is...

The root of any negative emotion is disturbance in the body's energy system.

There is no certainty of the method used however one thing is for certain: millions of people tap each day to get amazing results!

An overview of the EFT procedure

The EFT process is comprised of a series of steps that are simple:

First You select an incident, a feeling, behavior or an issue that needs to address - It is important to be particular and focussed on the sensation.

You then rate the intensity of your experience on a scale of to 10, and record the intensity for later comparison.

After that, you complete next the "Setup" and "Tap on it" by using the EFT procedure.

After that, you evaluate the intensity and decide if you'll need continue the tapping procedure to decrease the intensity even further.

Picking an issue to focus on

There are a myriad of issues you could tackle with EFT that go beyond migraine Headache symptoms. (For the reason of teaching EFT I'm using examples that are not related to migraines within this chapter. Later in the book, you will find a wealth of information about how to apply EFT Tapping for migraines.)

The most important thing is to be precise about the information and emotions you are addressing. You must reduce the issue down to parts, and take each part in turn to ensure maximum efficiency.

For instance an example "Fear of Flying" has several components or parts such as...

+ Claustrophobia

+ Fear of Heights

+ Not Being in Control

+ Leaving the Ground

+ The sensation of the sensation of

And even the smells of Jet engine exhaust...

...may be a part of the overall set of emotions with the tag "fear of flying."

The idea is that , after you break it into its constituent components, you begin by working on the specific component with the highest degree of discomfort or intensity.

Then, you can choose the term "summary description or label" for it

Some issues come with long descriptions. It is helpful to understand the lengthy description to be able to "tune-in" to all the details of the specific problem. This is an illustration for the "long description" of the problem.

"That time in the third grade when I was reading out loud in front of the class and I said the wrong word and I felt embarrassed because everyone laughed at me."

That will completely and precisely identify the issue that you are looking for by tapping.

However, using a lengthy description is a burden while tapping. We create the "summary description or label" to make use of as a shorthand to convey the issue as we tap. This "shorthand" is used during the process of setting up to represent the whole issue to be used for tapping. Additionally, it's utilized during tapping to help you stay focused on the issue, the way we have defined it in this particular session of taps. You are able to choose any "summary description or label" you like but the idea is to construct one that reflects your situation to keep your focus on the issue at hand.

In the case of the earlier example there are many ways to create an abbreviation for it. I could use the phrase, "Reading out loud embarrassment" If it was the most important thing for me. You could also write, "Class laughed at me in the 3rd grade" If that was the main aspect. Notice that I said "in the 3rd grade" since there could be other instances where my classmates laughed at me, however, I'd like to concentrate on this particular incident from the third grade. Another option is "Wrong word, reading out loud" It does not have necessarily be correct grammatically, or even correct.

Each of these phrases could actually refer to a different aspect of the problem. Sometimes , you might need the use of EFT to a variety of aspects of the issue to obtain an enormous amount of emotions out of the situation.

The concept behind"summary descriptions or labels "summary description or label" is to provide something that represents the issue for you, so that you can stay focussed on the issue at hand and not be able to shift to another topic without even noticing it. The shorthand is designed to focus your attention on the topic being dealt with instead of mentally jumping to other similar issues that might be in your mind. Similar items OFTEN occur when you are tapping. Just make a note of them, but then finish this round by using the initial focus for that period of tapping. It is possible to address the "new" items can be dealt with in another round of tapping should it be needed.

SUDS

It is beneficial to gauge the intensity of the object to be addressed to be able to more easily see the effect from tapping. To do this we take a measure of the intensity prior to tapping, and again immediately after tapping. We evaluate it by assigning it an SUDS rating.

SUDS are the acronym for Subjective Units of Distress Scale. It's an undefined scale ranging from 0 to 10, with 0 representing no intensity, while 10 being as strong as you can imagine it being.

Chapter 2: Forming The Setup Phrase

The first step in opening up about an issue is to recognize the issue! While this may sound simple, there's some nuances that many don't know about.

It is true that, without reason of your own, there can be a certain amount in the form of "Subconscious Self Sabotage" that operates beneath the surface, unnoticed and unnoticed. This is because there's a subconscious part of you that is refractory to overcoming the issue. This subconscious part might think that it's too "safe" to get over the issue, since it believes that being a victim of the issue protects the person in some fashion. In some cases, the subconscious part of you may believe there's a second benefit in being in the middle of an issue.

Let's take an example. For instance, suppose you were injured in your back and, as a result, you received disability payments. There is a sub-conscious part of you that thinks that if you did recover from your back injury, then you could lose your disability benefits. This is why you don't believe it would have been "safe" to get over the injury, which is why it isn't willing to let go. Although it could be true that you may lose your disability payment but that unconscious part is also being denied your conscious knowledge of the extent to which your life could be improved by overcoming the back injury and regaining your life even if you need to leave and take a job.

This and numerous others are part of the category of "Psychological Reversal." EFT provides a specific method of dealing with "Psychological Reversal," or PR, to increase the chances of success. It is done by completing"setup. "setup process" before actually beginning the tapping.

The Setup

The goal of the Setup is helping remove the "psychological reversal" that may be a result of the problem. The Setup involves tapping the Karate Chop spot on the hand's left side while repeating a certain "Setup Phrase."

"Karate Chop," also known as the "Karate Chop" spot or KC can be found on the side of your hand that lies between your small fingers and wrist. It's where you will strike something with the "Karate Chop." It isn't important which hand you tap with however I will always tap using the four fingers of the other hand.

The goal behind"Setup Phrase," or the "Setup Phrase" is to make the subconscious aware it is "even though you have the problem or issue, you really are OK." By telling the subconscious that you're okay even though you're having issues it's inclined to "get out of the way" and allow tapping to take the intended result.

The structure for the Setup Phrase is: "Even though I deeply and completely love and accept myself." In this instance, the"problem statement" can be a concise description of the issue or, as I often do,"summary descriptions or labels" as the "summary description or label" that we spoke about earlier.

One of the most important aspects to be aware of is being as precise as you can when defining the issue you'll have to address.

To begin the setup procedure, tap the Karate Chop spot while saying the Setup Phrase out loud...

+ "Even though I deeply and completely love and accept myself."

Repeat the Setup Phrase three times, while continuously tapping the Karate Chop Spot.

If we were to address the topic we talked about before it could be addressed as follows:

When you tap continuously at the Karate Chop spot, repeat three times in front of your eyes Three times.

+ "Even though the class laughed at me in the 3rd grade, I deeply and completely love and accept myself."

+ "Even though the class laughed at me in the 3rd grade, I deeply and completely love and accept myself."

+ "Even though the class laughed at me in the 3rd grade, I deeply and completely love and accept myself."

You could say "I deeply and completely love and accept myself," or, "I deeply and completely accept myself." Both are effective in signalling to the subconscious that you're okay.

Sometimes , people are incredibly unwilling to say, "I deeply and completely love and accept myself." The best thing to do is modify it to "I'm open to the possibility of deeply and completely loving and accepting myself...someday!" Most people who face difficulties with this can be "open for the possibilities ...."

Another thing I suggest doing is spending the time tapping out: "Even though I can't say that I deeply and completely love and accept myself, I deeply and completely love and accept myself anyway...or at least I'm open to that possibility someday!"

Tapping Process

The tapping takes place on specific areas of the body, while saying the "Reminder Phrase" to keep you "tuned in" to the problem being dealt with. It is the Reminder Phrase can be described as an example of the "summary description or label" we discussed earlier. It is a bilateral point, located on each side of your body or along the center lines of our bodies. They correspond to specific Acupuncture points. It is possible to tap on one side of your body, or tap on both sidesof the body, which is what I normally do. I usually tap with two fingers simultaneously because it covers a larger area and it doesn't require me to be as precise in hitting the exact area.

I usually tap around seven times at each location which is about the time it takes to repeat"THE" Reminder Phrase. The pressure of tapping should be firm but soft at least the same as what you use a keyboard while typing.

Tapping Locations

There are nine distinct areas that we'll need to tap on, as illustrated in the figure below.

They include:

+ The "Top" or Top of the Head.

And the "EB or Eyebrow located at the bottom, closest to the bridge of your nose.

And the "SE" or Side of the Eye is located in the bony ridge just beside the eye, not further back, on the temple's soft region.

+ + The "UE" or Under the Eye area located on the bony ridge, in line with the center of your eyes.

And The UN or under The Nose...is beneath the nose.

and the CH also known as the "Chin Spot" is the next one. It's known as"the "Chin spot" but it is actually beneath the lower lip.

And the CB also known as the Collar bone follows next location. It is located through taking your index finger, place it in what you call your "Adam's Apple" and then sliding it into the tiny U-shaped region at the base of your neck. Move your finger back and forth for around one inch, and you'll be sitting on your collarbone close to where it joins the sternum or breastbone.

+ The UA, also known as the Under Arm area is located to your right approximately 4 inches which is "a hand's width" below the arm pit.

We've also talked regarding the KC or "Karate Chop" spot which is located on the right side of the hand, between the base of the little finger and wrist.

To enhance this book, I made an animated video to show tapping locations more clearly than could be done using words and photos on their own. You can see the EFT Tapping Locations video here: http://tapping4.us/tappingspots. There is a complete video list and other web-based content in the Resources section.

We now know the location we'll tap, we can take a closer look through the EFT tapping procedure.

Chapter 3: Eft Protocol

The first step is decide on the problem to tackle, and then assign that issue a first score of 0-10.

Begin by tapping the Karate Chop spot while saying the Setup Phrase out loud, three times.

"Even though I deeply & completely love & accept myself."

Then, go through the sequence, saying"Reminder Phrase. "Reminder Phrase" as you tap on each spot. Tap on the Eyebrow, Side of the Eye, Under the Eye, Under the Nose, Chin, Collar Bone, Under the Arm, and Top of the Head.

I would suggest doing two or more taps at a time.

After you've completed several sessions of tapping and squeezing, take a deep breathe and give the problem a fresh SUDS rating.

In the end, evaluate the two SUDS ratingsto determine the next step.

When the 2nd SUDS rating is zero If the second SUDS rating is 0, then you might be completed with the "aspect or the issue." It is crucial to discover a method to test the issue in order to ensure that it is goneand there aren't any issues that you missed.

If your first SUDS score is less, do another set of tapping but this time , change the Reminder and Setup phrases to include "This is a reminder to keep this in place." ..."

The most recent Setup Phrase would be. "Even though I still have some of THIS REMAINING I deeply and completely love and accept myself."

It is important to recognize that there has been progress However, there's still a portion of the problem to be dealt with in another round of taps.

If the SUDS rating isn't changing, make sure you confirm that it's the same issue and you haven't gone to the next tapping subject without realizing. If you are able to see that this isn't the same problem, then think of it as an entirely new issue, then start with the same issue and tackle this new problem or issue by a fresh round of tapping.

If it is the same issue begin over and repeat your Setup Phrase out loud with EMPHASIS while tapping that Karate Chop spot. After that, you can tap through several rounds of EFT, before checking the SUDS once more.

It's not common for two SUDS rating higher than the previous one.

If that's the case, it's likely that you've really gotten into the issue more clearly or the more usual situation is that you've switched to a different issue or issue and not noticed the shift.

Sometimes, the shift is very subtle. If you encounter this scenario I would recommend that you record a detailed account of what is happening to allow for review following the next session of tapping. Make note of any differences in Location, Character or SUDS strength when in comparison to the description in writing of the issue to be addressed. I would also suggest performing numerous complete taps and repeating"Setup" and repeating the Setup Phrase with EMPHASIS before reviewing the SUDS rating.

If you're stuck, I suggest persevering. Try breaking your problem into smaller parts. Be more precise in your description of the problem, and work on it for a few days by doing multiple rounds of tapping each time.

If you're still stuck, I suggest consulting with someone who is an EFT practitioner. Perhaps you're not seeing something that they would be able to identify.

Basic steps to follow EFT tapping

Select an issue to make an "shorthand" description of it to use as a Reminder Phrase.

+ Add a SUDS rating.

• Setup the set-up by pressing the Karate Chop spot while saying out loud 3 times "Even though I have this I deeply and completely love and accept myself."

And then, while saying the Reminder Phrase in loud and then, perform a few sessions of tapping through all of them: EB, SE, UE, UN, CH, CB, UA, Top

And lastly breathe deeply and then give it a SUDS score again.

+ If there's some SUDS strength left, begin a second round by using the "Setup" Phrase and then using "this remaining" along with the Reminder Phrase.

EFT Tapping Examples

Below is a couple of most favorite EFT Tapping teaching demonstrations. They both provide a very powerful an experience that is personal to the kinds of shifts are created by EFT Tapping can bring about for us.

If you have access to chocolate (or another food item for which could trigger an intense SUDS desire for it) I would recommend you test the craving demonstration first. This exercise isn't going to "make you hate chocolate" but it could demonstrate the efficacy of EFT in shifting cravings. After you've witnessed that kind of shift it's much simpler to be confident in the EFT Tapping process , and it is much more likely to employ it to other areas of your life as well.

It is worth noting that chocolate is an Migraine trigger for certain individuals. Therefore, this demonstration might help in decreasing the desire for chocolate in those. If chocolate triggers migraine for you, you might think about changing the demonstration to not actually consuming or tasting the chocolate. The same demo of craving can be utilized with various Migraine trigger foods, too. Simply substitute the chocolate with the trigger food. Be sure to always be accountable for your actions as well as your overall health!

The second demonstration is a fantastic way of showing the ways that "stress and tension" can influence our bodies and limit our breathing . This is determined by "perceived lung capacity" during the demonstration. Even if you've already participated in the demonstration of craving, I still suggest taking part in the second demo. This is especially important when you are looking to treat physical issues like migraine headaches with the help of EFT tapping.

Craving Demo

If I am doing this type of teaching demonstration in front of an audience live I will usually bring some Hershey's Kisses chocolate that we make our "object of desire" so to say. I love using Kisses because they're small, are available in bulk, and they are individually wrapped, making it easier to distribute them to every member of the class. They're in addition "just chocolate" rather than "really good chocolate" so there's less anxiety among the class regarding "giving up their chocolate." If you possess some "just chocolate" available, take it right now, but don't open it or take a BITE yet! While you're at it get a piece of paper and a pencil or pencil to record your SUDS during the workout.

Step 1.) Increase your craving (craving) for chocolate!

Hold it in your palm and stare at it thinking about how great it tastes. Imagine unwrapping the chocolate and the sweet scent of the chocolate first affecting your senses. Imagine how wonderful it tastes as it melts inside your mouth. Do not eat it now, but try to think about it in your head.

Then write on that piece of paper how much you want the chocolate to satisfy - give it an "craving intensity" using the SUDS rating system you were taught about earlier.

You can now take a piece of chocolate. Place it in front of your nose and take some good whiffs of the scent of the delicious chocolate. Take note of how the urge for chocolate is making you feel now. It might be helpful to write down a few lines in a journal about the experience and the current level of SUDS.

Okay, now it's the time for you to take just a small bite of chocolate. Not a full bite, but only enough to taste the aroma that the chocolaty melts into your mouth with no chance of satisfying your desire to devour more.

Step 2.) Note down the SUDS level of your craving or desire to eat that chocolate.

Include a few words to express how you're experiencing about the desire to indulge in that chocolate!

Then, put the chocolate near where you will be able to take a look at it throughout the remaining demo sequence.

Step 3.) By tapping repeatedly at the Karate Chop (KC) spot and say: "Even though I crave chocolate, I deeply and completely accept and love myself. While I crave this chocolate, I truly and completely embrace myself and love me. Although I want the delicious chocolate I completely and deeply respect and love myself."

Step 4.) When you are looking at your chocolates, move your finger through the various locations while repeating"Crave that Chocolate!" Reminder Phrase "Crave That Chocolate!" at every point (to keep your attention on the actual craving.) Tap 5-7 times on each spot or tap repeatedly for the time it takes to say"Crave That Chocolate" Reminder Phrase, "Crave That Chocolate!"

+ Eyebrow (EB) - "Crave That Chocolate!"

+ Side of the eye (SE) - "Crave That Chocolate!"

+ Under the eye (UE) - "Crave That Chocolate!"

And Under the Nose (UN) + Under the nose (UN) "Crave That Chocolate!"

+ Chin (CH) - "Crave That Chocolate!"

+ Collar bone (CB) + Collar bone (CB) "Crave That Chocolate!"

+ Under the arm (UA) - "Crave That Chocolate!"

+ The top of head (Top) + Top of the head (Top) "Crave That Chocolate!"

Repeat the process of tapping the exact way : EB, SE, UE, UN, CH, CB, UA, Top and then saying "Crave That Chocolate!" and tap at each of the points.

Take your breath deeply, and let it go.

Step 5) Review the SUDS rating of your chocolate craving. Take an instant and then give the intensity of your desire for chocolate the SUDS score.

Take it out and sniff it. What is been the SUDS ratings changed? What is the difference? How does this different SUDS rating compare to the one you recorded prior to tapping? Do you think it is lower? If yes, how much? (In rare instances, it could have increased, which indicates it's because it's because you're "tuned into" the craving to a greater extent!) Take note of the sensation you feel when you gaze at the chocolate and consider eating it. Did the feeling change or altered in any way contrasted to the notes you made down? Try a second small sample, and observe what you can notice.

Note down the new SUDS rating, again, with any notes on the emotions you experienced.

6.) Another tap-round using "this left ..."

When you are you are looking at the chocolate, as you did during the initial round of tapping, perform another two sets of tapping. However, change your Setup Phrase along with the Reminder Phrase as illustrated below. It is important to acknowledge the fact that something has changed and also that there's an untapped SUDS concentration to be focused on in the next set of tapping.

When you are looking towards the chocolaty and making a continuous tap at the Karate Chop (KC) spot and say: "Even though I STILL desire chocolate I am incredibly and totally embrace myself and love my body. While I may still experience some of that chocolate craving I sincerely and completely respect and love myself. Although I still have some of that lingering lust for that yummy, delicious chocolate I deeply and completely respect and love myself."

Continue to stare at the chocolate while tapping the points, and then repeating "Remaining Chocolate Craving."

+ Eyebrow - "Remaining Chocolate Craving"

+ Side of the eye - "Remaining Chocolate Craving"

+ Under the eye - "Remaining Chocolate Craving"

And under the nose + Under the nose "Remaining Chocolate Craving"

+ Chin - "Remaining Chocolate Craving"

+ Collar bone "Remaining Chocolate Craving"

+ Under the arm - "Remaining Chocolate Craving"

+ Top of the head "Remaining Chocolate Craving"

Repeat the second repeat of tapping like the first time you did the first time - EB, SE, UE, UN, CH, CB, UA, Top and then saying "Remaining Chocolate Craving" and tapping each of them.

Step 7) You should check your SUDS score for the chocolate desire. Consider it for some time and then give the intensity of the desire for chocolate the SUDS score.

Then, pick it up and smell it. Is been the SUDS rate changed? What does the different SUDS rating compare to the one you recorded prior to tapping? Do you think it is lower? If so, how much? Take note of the feelings you experience when you take a look at the chocolate and consider eating it. Did the sensation shift or altered in any way contrasted to the notes you made down? Take one small bite, and then observe what you feel.

Record this new SUDS rating, again, with any notes on the feelings you observed.

For those who take part in this exercise, it will result in a significant change in the SUDS level of craving. There will be a few confused stares in the room while they attempt to understand the changes they have experienced "from this silly tapping thing" that they have just done!

If you are determined to experience the complete EFT Tapping Experience, continue to repeat the steps 6 and 7 until your desire for chocolate is satisfied to a SUDS score of zero. I'd suggest you try a few more times of tapping, using the Setup, so that are able to experience the thrill of achieving the SUDS level of zero.

One of the things most shocking for the majority of people is the change in the flavor of the chocolate. For me the first time I attempted that with hershey's Kisses I observed the what I called a "more chemical taste" than I was noticing initially.

In a quick aside, Gary Craig also noticed what he refers to as "the apex effect" occurs occasionally. Sometimes, people undergo a series of tapping on something that's distressing them emotionally, such as trauma or fear and, at the end of the tapping session, after their SUDS have dropped to zero, or even close to zero, they'll "wave off the results" of the tapping. Sometimes they'll say "the tapping distracted me from the problem," or "well, it wasn't really that much of a problem to begin with in the first place!" It's incredible to witness. This is one of reasons I always make sure that when I work with someone who is new to EFT Tapping that they write in their own handwriting the SUDS score at every stage. It's much harder for them to "deny the results" that this way! It's not to scold them over it, but rather to demonstrate the results in black-and white, so that they don't lose sight of the opportunities which EFT Tapping presents in their lives.

To enhance this book, I made an online video to show an EFT Chocolate Craving Demo more clear than could be accomplished using just words and photos. You can see the video for the Chocolate Craving Demo here: http://tapping4.us/chocolatedemo. You can access a comprehensive list of videos as well as other content on the internet in the Resources section.

Chapter 4: Breathing Demo

This EFT Tapping for Constricted Breathing demonstration is unique because it will clearly illustrate the connection to EFT Tapping as well as the body's response to physical. Although this demonstration can be very eye-opening for a lot of people due to the amount of shift they observe while others might only be able to notice a tiny amount of change. The demo is best done in a setting with a group in which a group of people are able to share their experiences with the workout and the degree of change they see. It's worth taking part in this exercise even if it is alone.

Another intriguing aspect of this demonstration is that it can "peel away layers of intensity" from the general issue and help you remember specific events or to be able to explain the problem more clearly to be able to address it by more EFT tapping.

The breathing demonstration includes being bent around, and if are suffering from Migraine symptoms You might want to return to this exercise later and test it after Migraine symptoms have gone away.

Step 1.) "Stretch your lungs." The goal is to do three deep breaths the lungs stretch little before setting the basis in the practice. It is not necessary to be hyperventilating Take your time and spread your deep breaths over a few minutes.

A way to accomplish the same is standing up and exhale as you bend forward to drop your arms to the floor. Inhale deeply while you stand up , and then raise your arms out and up to make sure they are over your head. This will allow you to expand your ribcage and stretch it and permit the full expansion of your lungs.

Step 2.) Once you've extended your lungs as long as they will allow and you are ready to take another deep breath. Then, evaluate what you feel is the "deepness of your breath" on a scale ranging from 0 to 10 where 10 is the best estimation (or estimation) of what your max lung capacity is. Make sure you write the results down on a piece of paper for later comparison. Values assigned generally range in between three and nine during this particular portion of the test. (It is important to remember that a lot of people who assign an incorrect value of 10 for this initial measurement, discover that after many sessions of EFT Tapping they must give an end-of-day value between 12 and 15 due to their assessment of the increased breathing capacity.)

Step 3.) Then, prepare to perform multiple rounds of EFT tapping using a setup phrase such as, "Even though I have constricted breathing ..." or "Even even though I'm able to breathe in eight inches ..." for example.

Take note of the part below, where I state "...fill the lungs up to the sound of an 8, ..."

replace the number you got from step 2 for 8 in that sentence.

Also, as you continue to tap to the Karate Chop (KC) spot and say: "Even though I have constricted breathing I deeply and totally respect and love myself. Even though I suffer from constricted breathing, I sincerely and completely respect and love myself. Even though I'm constricted in my breathing and can limit my breathing with 8or so, I truly and totally love and accept myself."

Step 4.) Begin to tap on each of the points , while repeating"Reminder" Phrase "Constricted Breathing" at each location. Tap five to seven times in each area or tap until you can say"Constricted Breathing" as the Reminder Phrase.

+ Eyebrow - "Constricted Breathing"

+ Side of the eye - "Constricted Breathing"

+ Under the eye - "Constricted Breathing"

and under the nasal bridge + Under the nose "Constricted Breathing"

+ Chin - "Constricted Breathing"

+ Collar bone "Constricted Breathing"

+ Under the arm - "Constricted Breathing"

+ Top of the head "Constricted Breathing"

After you've completed this tap and taking a deep breath similar to the way you had before, and evaluate your "deepness of your breath" on a scale of 0-10, then note it down and compare it with the original measurement.

Then, repeat a second cycle of tapping exactly like this: EB, SE, UE, UN, CH, CB, UA, Top and bottom while saying "I can only fill my lungs to an 8" while tapping at each of the points.

+ Eyebrows + Eyebrow "I can only fill my lungs to an 8"

+ Eye side + Side of the eye "I can only fill my lungs to an 8"

And under your eye + Under the eye "I can only fill my lungs to an 8"

And under the nose + Under the nose "I can only fill my lungs to an 8"

Chin + "I can only fill my lungs to an 8"

+ Collar bone "I can only fill my lungs to an 8"

and under the arm "I can only fill my lungs to an 8"

+ Top of the head "I can only fill my lungs to an 8"

After you've completed the second set in tapping your feet, do a full breath, and then evaluate what you consider to be the "deepness of your breath" on a scale of 0-10. then note it down and then compare it to the initial assessment.

Then, repeat a third cycle of tapping exactly the same way, EB, SE, UE, UN, CH, CB, UA, Top as you alternate between repeating "Constricted Breathing" and "I can only fill my lungs to an 8" while you tap at each of the points. (Alternating the words you're saying keeps you engaged and focused, and helps to alleviate some of the boredom that is caused by repeating the same phrase over and over again.)

+ Eyebrow - "Constricted Breathing"

Side of the eye + Side of the eye "I can only fill my lungs to an 8"

+ Under the eye - "Constricted Breathing"

and under the nose + Under the nose "I can only fill my lungs to an 8"

+ Chin - "Constricted Breathing"

+ Collar bone "I can only fill my lungs to an 8"

+ Under the arm - "Constricted Breathing"

+ The top of the head "I can only fill my lungs to an 8"

After you've completed the third time of tapping, take a full, deep breath, in the same way you did prior to tapping and then evaluate how you feel about the "deepness of your breath" on a scale of 0-10. take note of it and then compare it to your first and second round evaluations.

Many people are somewhat shocked to learn that their lung capacity has increased in the demonstration. Many people may even be able to provide "interesting answers" to questions such as "What does this constricted breathing remind you of?" "When in your past did your feel constricted or smothered?" "If there was an emotional reason for this constricted breathing, what might it be?" In most cases, they will open up new areas of exploration and EFT tapping. It's usually beneficial to note down those memories, thoughts and thoughts that manifest themselves in these scenarios.

They often provide significant clues regarding crucial emotional issues that can be dealt with using EFT Tapping.

Online video example

While the internet is ever changing, at the time of publication of this book you can find a video of a group "constricted breathing" demonstration on Gary Craig's website through this link: http://tapping4.us/breathing.

Troubleshooting suggestions for common problems when using EFT Tapping

EFT Tapping could be used to treat a vast range of issues that you face in your daily life. Below are some of the most frequent problems and tips on how to deal with these issues.

Too general

One of the primary reasons for difficulty producing results using EFT Tapping is being too general in the definition of the issue. Try to find the SPECIFIC sensation and the location it is situated in your body, particularly when it comes to physical problems.

It could be an individual event (or memories of an or a specific event) which is bothering you. Do not lump everything into the same category. Make them distinct and discuss them individually.

In the process of losing track of the issue

One of the issues that comes with EFT Tapping is that things change so rapidly that it is difficult to remember precisely what caused the issue. I suggest writing down the precise details of the issue that you are trying to address during each session of tapping. This helps you remain focussed on the specific issue and assists you in identifying subtle changes that may occur. This is particularly relevant for physical problems, and can help you recognize the signs that things are changing when the "chase the pain." Sometimes, it appears to be that SUDS intensities are the same however when you look closer, you'll observe that the character has changed, from acute pain to a an ache that is dull, for instance. This is definitely a change and is a the beginning of resolution.

Speak the truth to be able to address the root of the problem.

Don't "sugar coat it," or downplay it or do anything to be politically correct in the way you define the problem. Express what you feel and make sure you use your own words! Do not use the phrase, "I don't like to exercise," when you are feeling that "Exercise is a pain in the ass!"

You're trying to tune to the actual issue so you can take action and let it go! But it's impossible to focus on it when you're not expressing that "like it is" and in a manner that is consistent with your feelings!

The skipping of steps

Another reason for difficulties is not completing the steps. If you're not tapping the Karate Chop spot (KC) and using the Setup Phrase and you're experiencing slow or have no progress, return, include the Setup Phrase and use it with a strong voice when tapping the KC. Be sure to be precise in the description of the problem!

A solution to an undefined, poorly defined issue that isn't clearly defined or well-defined

Another problem that can be present is the difficulty of the problem or being able to pinpoint a specific area to tap. Be aware that you are able to tap into the sensations inside your body, which comes up whenever you think of the problem.

You can also press "Even although I'm not certain the reason why I'm feeling like this ..." and "Even when I'm not able to discern the problem ..." or anything similar to that.

EFT Tapping on a Page

Applying EFT Tapping For Fast Migraine Headache Relief

Disclaimer: The information provided in this article is intended for informational purposes only. The information isn't medical and isn't to be regarded to be medical advise. You should consult with a qualified doctor prior to making any decision based on this information. Check out the disclaimer at beginning of this book for further details.

How to utilize this section

This section delved into the specifics of how to apply EFT Tapping especially to treat Migraine Headache manifestations.

If you're suffering from a Migraine Headache is beginning today...

...then I'd recommend you immediately go over to "Migraine Tapping Fast Start" section and follow the instructions by doing the exercises shown in the section.

If you don't exhibit Migraine symptoms at the moment...

...then I would recommend reading through this article and then taking the exercises until you are aware of the methods of EFT tapping to treat an Migraine Headache prior to the next session begins.

Beginning by Migraine Headache TFT tapping

Many ways EFT tapping for Migraine Headache effects is similar to treating any other physical symptom using EFT tapping. The idea is to concentrate on the symptoms and then tap. The process guides you through the reduction of symptoms to completion by observing the SUDS intensity, character and location of the symptoms. This is done while "chasing the pain" as it is usually described.

Utilizing SUDS, Character and the location for guidance during your tap

In the earlier part of this book, SUDS refers to Subject units of distress scale. It is the scale of 0-10, which is arbitrary, is utilized in order to "measure" the intensity of the symptoms. Zero refers to zero level of intensity, while 10 refers for "being as intense as you can imagine it to be." When you use the SUDS for assessing the intensity prior to and following sessions of tapping you can better assess and quantify the changes that occur.

A "Character of a symptom" can include descriptors like Sharp Dull, Throbbing Stabbing, Achy dizziness, Nausea and any similar descriptive term that can be used to describe. It's not exactly the Character that's crucial however, it's the change in Character that can affect the process. You are free to select whatever phrases define what you consider to be the "Character" of the symptom for you, but make sure you know what this definition means for you to be able to be aware of the changes.

Location is among the most simple factors to determine. It's often the case that one can identify what is the "exact" Location of a discomfort or symptom on the body's surface - "behind and slightly above my left eye socket," for instance. However, it's not the exact location that is important but the change in the symptoms you're noticing that directs the course of action.

I often suggest to those who are only getting started with EFT Tapping to record their SUDS and Character and location information to ensure that they are sure of the details of the "starting conditions." This information can be particularly useful when they revisit to review the changes after the initial and subsequent round of tapping. It eliminates any doubts and can help build trust in tapping as well as knowledge.

Example Tapping Script Walk-Through

Here is an example of a tapping script walk-through of the entire procedure, including the factors that determine the decision and the criteria used to decide about what to do next. This is an abbreviated version of what you might encounter, meaning that you might require additional rounds of tapping beyond what are listed here. If you follow this guideline, it will be easy for you to know exactly what you need to do and how you can make decisions on how to go with the process, in accordance with your SUDS Character and the location of your particular condition and symptoms.

In this case, we'll presume that it's middle of the afternoon when you realize that you are suffering from the first sign of Migraine Headache. It's been a busy day during lunch, and you were focusing on various tasks that demanded your attention completely, so you didn't notice the initial signs of the disease's precursor.

SUDS, Character, & Location - Initial Assessment

You've just experienced a brief interruption in your focus and you have noticed the following signs:

A dull, throbbing pain just behind and below the inside that lies above your left eye, with an SUDS rating of five. The muscles of your scalp with a general SUDS of 3 but it's stronger to the left, above your ear , with an SUDS rating of 4 in this area. Your vision may be somewhat "off" but full-blown auras aren't yet happening, so the SUDS is 2.

It is important to note it is three distinct symptoms descriptions here : The tension, pain and the visual symptoms. The most affluent SUDS score is 5 for pain, and that's the one to concentrate on first.

Chapter 5: Setting Up Phrase As Well As Kc Tapping

The above description of the SUDS Character, SUDS and Location is quite long, therefore it's not practical to repeat it each time as the Setup Phrase or Reminder Phrase. Therefore it is possible to create the shorthand version. Since we'll concentrate on the pain during the initial tapping sessions, we'll use the description that is short, "This 5 throbbing eye pain" to indicate the more detailed and longer description.

You can begin your EFT Tapping process by tapping repeatedly on the"karate chop" (or "karate chop" spot, (see diagram) as you repeat three times the Setup Phrase, three times, "Even though I have this 5 throbbing eye pain, I deeply and completely love and accept myself."

Tapping into the points

Then you'll tap each location as you repeat that Reminder Phrase "This 5 throbbing eye pain." (Tap approximately five to seven times at each location or continuously until you can repeat"This 5 throbbing eye pain." Reminder Phrase.)

+ Eyebrows + Eyebrow "This 5 throbbing eye pain."

+ Eye side + Side of the eye "This 5 throbbing eye pain."

And under your eye + Under the eye "This 5 throbbing eye pain."

and under the eye + under the nose "This 5 throbbing eye pain."

+ Chin + Chin "This 5 throbbing eye pain."

+ Collar bone "This 5 throbbing eye pain."

And under your arm "This 5 throbbing eye pain."

+ The top of the head "This 5 throbbing eye pain."

Then , do another cycle of tapping exactly in the same manner - EB, SE, UE, UN, CH, CB, UA, Top with the words "This 5 throbbing eye pain" and tapping every point.

Now , take your breath deeply, and let it go.

Character, SUDS, and Reassessment of location

It is time to review the SUDS, Character and location and location of symptoms. In this case, we'll take the assumption that the description that is represented by "This 5 throbbing eye pain" is not altered However, the intensity has decreased from an SUDS rating of 5 to a.

It changed

Since the description of the symptoms has been the same, but it is evident that the SUDS intensity has diminished and we'd like to do a second EFT tapping session with the latest phrase, Reminder "This REMAINING throbbing eye pain." In this situation, we would like to recognize that SUDS intensity has decreased but there's still remaining pain that must be taken care of.

Tapping through the points Round 2.

In the next round of tapping, we'll make a smart decision and leave out the Setup-KC Tapping section as it's only required approximately 40 percent of the time, and we did it before the initial session of taps (which I highly recommend!)

Tapping into those parts...

+ Eyebrows + Eyebrow "This remaining throbbing eye pain."

+ Eye side + The side of the eye "This remaining throbbing eye pain."

and under the eyes + Under the eye "This remaining throbbing eye pain."

and under the eye "This remaining throbbing eye pain."

+ Chin + Chin "This remaining throbbing eye pain."

+ Collar bone "This remaining throbbing eye pain."

and under the arm "This remaining throbbing eye pain."

+ Top of the head "This remaining throbbing eye pain."

Then , do another repeat of tapping in like this: EB, SE, UE, UN, CH, CB, UA, Top with the words "This remaining throbbing eye pain" and tap at every point.

Now , take your breath deeply, then let it go.

Character, SUDS and Location reassessment following round 2.

It is time to reevaluate your SUDS and Character and location that the signs are manifesting. You can take a look and note that the SUDS severity is still an average of 3.

It didn't change , so what changed?

This is a place where many people get confused. The last paragraph didn't provide any specifics in the way it was measured but the SUDS intensity was still a 3. Many people are unable to grasp this in everyday life. They'll notice the overall SUDS severity of their "most intense symptom" but not realize that it's not the same as the symptom discussed in the previous tapping session.

One way to stop this for happening is to record the specifics of the specific symptom you're tapping for a specific session of tapping. So you can go back and review exactly where you began and what you were focusing on during the period of taps.

In this illustration, we'll presume that "throbbing eye pain" SUDS intensity has decreased to 0 1 or 2 that makes "scalp muscle tension" the most severe symptom with 3. This is shadowing"throbbing eyes "throbbing eye pain" so it's not being seen as a symptom.

For this second session of tapping, we'll presume it is the case that "throbbing eye pain" is not as obvious because it's "hiding behind" the "scalp muscle tension." The eye pain can persist to decrease when you tap other signs. If not, as the severity of other symptoms decrease, it could be resurfacing for further tapping focus.

Tapping through the points Tapping through the points - Round 3

Because we are experiencing a different issue that we did not experience in the previous tapping session, we'll begin by doing tapping the Setup along with KC tapping. Tap constantly onto your KC as you repeat your Setup Phrase, three times, "Even though I have this scalp muscle tension, I deeply and completely love and accept myself."

Then, by tapping on all the lines...

+ Eyebrows + Eyebrow "This scalp muscle tension."

+ Eye side + Side of the eye "This scalp muscle tension."

and under the eyes + Under the eye "This scalp muscle tension."

• Under the nose + Under the nose "This scalp muscle tension."

+ Chin + Chin "This scalp muscle tension."

+ Collar bone "This scalp muscle tension."

and under the arm + Under the arm "This scalp muscle tension."

+ The top of the scalp + the top of the head "This scalp muscle tension."

Then , do another repeat of tapping like the first time - EB, SE, UE, UN, CH, CB, UA, Top with the words "This remaining scalp muscle tension" and tap at every point.

Take an inhale, then let it go.

Character, SUDS and Reassessment of the location following round 3.

It is the time to reevaluate the SUDS, character, and location that the symptoms manifest. In this instance you will be able to see that each manifestation has diminished by SUDS intensity. Although every manifestation may not be reduced to zero, it is possible to declare it to be complete. However, I would recommend that you continue the EFT tapping applying it to each sign until it is at a level that it is feasible. At some point, SUDS levels of 1 or less will dissipate in the course of time. But why do you risk it when a couple of minutes of tapping might end it.

To enhance this book, I've created an instructional video that demonstrates how to do the Migraine EFT Tapping Script Walk Through in a more clear way than it could be by using photos and words alone. You can see the Migraine EFT Tapping Script Walk Through video here: http://tapping4.us/migrainewalkthru. You can access a comprehensive list of videos as well as other web-based content under the section Resources.

Important things to look out for...

...especially when your progression is slow

Concentrate on the sensation

One of the key factors to tapping the right chord is to be focused on the sensations and feelings. It's often simpler to just observe and evaluate what is happening instead of stopping to contemplate it to understand the specifics. The purpose of evaluating the SUDS, Character and Location is to build an understanding of the context with that you can observe and gauge the shifts happening.

Add Setup Phrase

Sometimes, I decide not to perform the setup and KC tapping prior to each round of tapping. It's an intentional risk that is borne of the experience. The most important thing to keep in mind is that if you're "not making progress" as described by SUDS reduction, you should include the Setup and KC tap back in Be sure to use the Setup Phrase with insistence! It's incredible what a change that can be made.

This is the conclusion of the Example Tapping Walk-Through of Scripts.

Migraine Tapping Fast Start

This section assumes that you're completely responsible for your well-being and self-care and have consulted a licensed medical professional before beginning applying this method. EFT Tapping methods described here.

If you've read the previous chapters of this book including the disclaimer and also completed the exercises, then you've got an understanding of the content that will be covered here and the motivation behind the concept.

When this is not the initial part of the book you're reading, review the Disclaimer page prior to proceeding. The main point is that you have to be accountable for yourself and your well-being and health. It is assumed that you've examined with a certified medical professional prior to participating with this EFT Tapping described below. If this is otherwise, you should proceed only after you've completed your check-up.

Step 1.) Take note of the location of the, the character, and the SUDS strength for your Migraine Headache signs. (Example of this is a dull, sharp pain that is located slightly in the middle and over the outside part of your eye. It has an intensity rating of five on the SUDS scale of 0-10.)

Step 2.) As you tap your (KC) Karate Chop spot (see the diagram below) speak out loudly, "Even though I have these Migraine Headache symptoms, I deeply and completely love and accept myself," and at the point that you are saying "these Migraine Headache symptoms" stop for a few seconds before focusing on the exact location, character and SUDS strength in the manifestations. It is important to be clear on what you intend to change in the process of "looking at" the way it is now.

Complete the KC Tapping step three times.

Step 3.) Tap on each of the locations shown in the diagram, while saying your Reminder Phrase "these Migraine Headache symptoms." (Tap around five to seven times at each point or tap repeatedly until it takes to repeat"this Migraine Headache symptom." Reminder Phrase.)

+ Eyebrows "These Migraine Headache symptoms."

+ The side of the eye + Side of the eye "These Migraine Headache symptoms."

And under your eye + Under the eye "These Migraine Headache symptoms."

and under the nasal bridge "These Migraine Headache symptoms."

+ Chin + Chin "These Migraine Headache symptoms."

+ Collar bone "These Migraine Headache symptoms."

And under your arm "These Migraine Headache symptoms."

+ Top of the head "These Migraine Headache symptoms."

Do a second repeat of tapping in like this: EB, SE, UE, UN, CH, CB, UA, Top with the words "These Migraine Headache symptoms" and tap at each of the points.

Now , take an inhale, then let it go.

Step 4.) Reevaluate the location of the, Character, and the severity in your Migraine Headache manifestations and compare them with your initial assessment.

If the Character and the Location exactly the same however the SUDS intensity has decreased Then repeat a handful of EFT tapping sessions and substitute your Reminder Phrase using "These REMAINING Migraine Headache symptoms." Follow up with Step 4 to figure out what you should do next.

If the Location or the character has changed, you should go back step 1 to treat it as the "new" version of the symptoms of migraine. The idea is that you're "chasing the pain" and making several cycles of tapping every "version" of the pain in order to lessen your SUDS intensity. If you observed a shift in the character or location this is considered to be as a "new version" of the symptoms and you should begin at the beginning of Step 1. It is considered improvement since it is the case that symptoms from "old version" of the symptoms are no longer present (or at the very least, are no anymore as prevalent as those of the "new version").

Keep trying with "chase the symptoms" by performing multiple cycles of EFT tapping for the "new set of symptoms" that is defined by changes in the location or Nature of symptoms. If you find that it's simply the SUDS intensity that has changed, just go through the points again with "this left ..." along with your Reminder Phrase.

After a few taps at the same time, you will likely discover you've found that your Migraine Headache symptoms have either) drastically diminished and/or B) not significantly changed or not changed at all. In either case, it is important to keep in mind that you've agreed to assume full responsibility for your well-being, and it might be time to look at alternatives to treatment options that can help you move towards Migraine symptoms relief.

If your symptoms appear to have diminished but aren't "completely gone" then I would suggest doing a few sessions of EFT tapping employing techniques such as the "chase the symptom" technique until they're nearly gone. It is important to keep in mind that if your symptoms begin to return you could repeat the same tapping process for these symptoms as well.

When I first assisted a friend of mine who was suffering from her migraine, she experienced quick relief with EFT tapping, however she was required to do additional tapping each time the symptoms began to return that day. The first time she began tapping was immediately after she was aware of the signs and didn't sit around waiting for their SUDS strength to rise. I'd recommend this same approach for you.

To add more information to this book, I've created an instructional video that demonstrates what I call the Migraine Tapping Fast Start more easily than you can by using only words and pictures. You can see the Migraine Tapping Fast Start video here: http://tapping4.us/migrainefaststart. You can access a comprehensive video list and other web-based content within the Resource section.

This completes this section "Migraine Tapping Fast Start" section.

Persistence is the power behind it.

Sometimes, things aren't working out as you would expect they will. This could be the case with EFT Tapping too, just like everything else. The "worst" that will happen is that you could lose a bit of time tapping on an issue or symptom, but it does not seem to change after three or four minutes of your finest tapping technique. If this happens this is happening, I'd recommend a few suggestions. (As previously stated the first thing is that you have to be accountable for your health and take action that is best for you and your circumstances.) My first suggestion is to revisit the process and attempt it in the future. Sometimes, that's all it'll require, just a new approach for a new day. Another option is to seek the assistance of someone else, a "tapping buddy" who is "outside" of the problem or issue. They may be able to offer new perspectives and highlight things you may have missed or did not notice. I've seen that happen in the occasion for me.

The key is to keep applying EFT tapping in your daily life. As mentioned in the other sections of this book EFT tapping is a solution to various circumstances and issues as well as people have excellent results applying it to their lives. The persistence in applying it to your daily life is likely to bring about the same result.

Chapter 6: Use Of Eft Tapping To Treat Migraine Headache Triggers

A single of Gary Craig's most important areas of teaching is the connection between emotional states and physical manifestations. It doesn't take for long to find examples of this link within our personal lives. It doesn't appear to be too far to contemplate the possibility that emotions could constitute one of the major factors that can trigger migraine symptoms. The first step in altering the situation is to increase awareness of potential triggers and identify the ones that are present throughout our day.

Recognizing triggers

For the sake of simplicity Let's divide the possible Migraine triggers down into two parts that are physical triggers and emotional triggers. It is important to note that there is a wide range of possible causes of Migraine symptoms. It could be due to a sensitization to environmental or food sources or deficiency in nutrition or hormonal imbalance or something more serious, such as an endocrine tumor. It is crucial to take responsibility for yourself and seek advice from a certified health professional.

Physical Triggers

Physical triggers can include things like environmental or food triggers. Your physician is likely to provide a list of possible triggers. These could include foods that contain preservatives (e.g. Nitrates, nitrates MSG) alcohol, the red wine industry, as well as coffee tea and cola, as well as artificial sweeteners, as well as specific food items like chocolate, aged cheeses citrus fruits or peanut butter, as well as nuts and salty foods. Environmental triggers could include smoke or chemicals, odors and smogs scents and fragrances or weather, as well as the barometric pressure and temperature.

Some of these variables are definitely out of our hands such as the weather however others are more within our control, for instance, the food choices. In any situation, there's likely to be some benefit in knowing what could trigger symptoms of Migraine for you.

It might seem odd to consider trying this however there are instances where people have tried EFT tapping with the intent to change food or environmental, sensitivities , and have experienced positive results.

I'm aware that I've personally tried EFT Tapping to create shifts in unanticipated areas. There was a period that was about a decade ago, when I was lactose intolerant and it manifested in the form of stomach swelling. I was in a position to use EFT Tapping in the course of time, while looking at a variety of possibilities, and greatly decreased the severity of my "apparent lactose intolerance." Although I cannot assure that the same result to you personally, I do hope that this article has enthralled you enough to look at ways to use EFT Tapping to this kind of situation in your own daily life.

My reason for sharing that tale with you is the fact that we are smart organic machines that can change and shift in unexpected ways, depending on your physical, and "emotional environment."

The emotional triggers

The emotional triggers that cause migraine symptoms might not be as obvious at first glance as the triggers that environmental causes are. But if we look at the many ways our bodies react in response to stressful situations, they become evident

Stress

Stress is a contributory factor in the Migraine trigger in a variety of ways. The medical profession has realized that not just can high levels of stress cause migraines, but it's often the cumulative effects of stress that triggers Migraines too. On the other side, there is evidence that stress-related letting down on vacations, weekends or even after the completion of a difficult project could cause migraines.

EFT Tapping is utilized frequently, and especially in a routine manner to lower the stress levels of your life which can reduce the chance of developing symptoms of migraine. Start tap on "...all the stress ..." that's quite general, and after several sessions of tapping that further, pay attention to more specific aspects like"Oh, "...my manager is urging to make this happen ...", "...I cannot imagine having to bail them out and make this right yet again!" or even "...I cannot believe that they're an idiot! Do they not recognize what the issue really is?" Simply choose the phrase that best describes the source of your stress, and begin tapping!

Sometimes, simply speaking to the stress-inducing thoughts that are going through your mind, while tapping on them continuously and speaking them out loud will reduce your stress levels. If you're like many people, then you likely have a tendency to to "bitch and complain" about issues that are bothersome for you or causing you stress. The good thing is that by speaking those thoughts loudly as you tap, you are likely to experience a change in the intensity of the thoughts. It could take longer than a few minutes, particularly if there are a lot however, in the end when I practice this I feel my stress levels to be significantly decreased, at minimum for a short time. Because I'm convinced that this is a highly effective strategy, I've created an internet site that focuses on this approach. You can find it at http://www.TapAndBitch.com and when you enter your name and email address in the box in the upper right-hand corner of the site, you will be sent access to a free 23-

minute video that I created called The EFT Quick Start Video Learning System. I highly recommend you take a look. (Not to offend or cause offending however "TapAndComplain.com" simply doesn't have the same impact, and isn't quite as memorable.)

An important note to those who adhere to The Law Of Attraction so they don't tend to be focused upon "negative things," but instead, they should maintain their perspective and keep it positive. As the creator of The Secret For Law Of Attraction video-based training program that is available on Amazon.com I can say that If your "focus on the negative" for long enough to use EFT tapping as well as "release the energy you have around it" you will have a much better chance of success in implementing applying the Law Of Attraction! This is because you're likely to notice that the thoughts and emotions that you've tapped aren't surfacing frequently.

With tapping, you've "taken the emotional charge off" the things you are thinking about and, as a result, you will are less occupied with them, and consequently less time trying to remind your self not to "not think about them or put your attention there," because they do not occur! Think about this two possibilities: On the one side, you might spend a few minutes "focusing on the negative thing" while tapping on it, so that it's released. This could result in the negative thoughts "visiting" you less, and a lower level of intensity. However, you might spend a minute every daily "accidentally" thinking about the negative until you realize that you are doing it and shift your attention to something positive. What is the average amount of time you expect to accumulate over one month for each situation? I'm willing to place my money into tapping.

Try it out and I'm sure you'll be surprised.

Stress induced by anticipation

Sometimes, we may work ourselves to a stressful state when we anticipate an event in the near future which we anticipate to be difficult. Such a situation could cause a surge in stress, and could trigger symptoms of migraine.

The application of EFT Tapping to situations that you're afraid might happen, (since it hasn't occurred yet, you aren't sure if it is going to happen) can be an effective way to not just decrease your stress, but gain a more resilient situation where you are able to anticipate and respond to the situation rather than reacting to your anxieties.

It is possible to tap issues such as "...I do not know what's about to happen ..." as well as "...I'm concerned that (fill-in-the-blank) will occur ..." and "...I do not exactly what I should do in the event that (fill-in-the-blank) occurs ..." or something similar to that. The act of reciting it while tapping the areas will lower your stress levels at the moment.

On the other hand, this could be that it is the possibility of a Migraine trigger. It doesn't need to mean "negative stress." It could be the stress that comes from the anticipation of something positive as well. The body might not be able distinguish between these two situations, and tapping could be helpful in both cases.

People, Anger, Power & Control

Without going too deeply into this, I'll let you know that it will not be uncommon to have people who live in your home who "trigger Migraine symptoms." If we looked deeper into this, I could possibly make a convincing argument to support the idea that the Migraine symptoms might be your body's attempt to "protect itself" while keeping you from any "bad" situation.

Let's take this example as an illustration. Let's say that in a hypothetical scenario you and your mother-in law aren't getting together well...at all! Let's say that each time you go to visit with her, or even present in her presence the it's like things "go badly" to put it simply. Every time you detect that you could be near her, your stress level increases. As the date gets closer the stress levels continue to increase. In this type of situation it is possible that symptoms of migraine begin to appear just before it's time to leave to go to the event, thereby hindering your attendance. If you observe that this pattern is occurring often, it is likely the body's intelligence "found a way to keep you safe" by not interacting with your mother-in law at the celebration. It's obvious that this is not a perfect example, however it does illustrate the idea.

Consider shifting the situation to the point where the main feeling is one of anger. The more intense anger, the greater the stress levels. A similar process could occur.

The reason I'm telling this story is so that I can give you the chance to view things with a new lens. There might be (and frequently is!) more happening beneath the surface than is apparent to the eye. Tapping can be an effective instrument to address various issues that arise in your daily life, and to reduce your stress levels also. But to take your tapping abilities to a higher level, which gives you more power and are able to shift things that have the root cause You must develop the "detective skills" to help to uncover the deeper causes.

In this book, I've attempted to provide you with some aspects of the "tricks of the trade" and techniques I employ to obtain faster and better outcomes with EFT Tapping , for both my clients as well as for myself.

Tapping to triggers

In the previous sections, I've offered different suggestions for the best way to tackle issues, as well as some suggestions for specific words. They are a great "jumping off point" to begin your journey of tapping to find triggers. One of the most important aspects to keep in mind is to continue tapping and exploring all possible possibilities to find "things to tap on" which could bring relief. The most perseverance is your most reliable friend in this situation. It might take a while and some digging to discover the source of the problem so that you can get it resolved at its root.

In addition to the concepts and suggestions inside this guide, further sources that can help you on this journey are available in the resource section towards the rear of the book.

Tapping FAQ

In the hopes that readers will not skim through this section, I've added in anticipation of people skipping around, I have included the "check with a qualified medical practitioner" statement in many answers. There are a few additional repetitions of statements within this section, so that each answer are able to stand on their own and be fully complete.

Chapter 7: Do I Have To Talk With My Physician Prior To Making Use Of Eft Tapping?

Like everything health-related it is recommended to consult with a licensed medical professional prior to starting any new program. This applies to EFT Tapping as well. There is an increasing amount of study-based evidence published in peer reviewed scholarly journals, the medical community hasn't "officially endorsed" the use of EFT Tapping. One example of this of this is the The Dr. David Feinstein's Acupoint Stimulation for the Treatment of Psychological Disorders Evidence of Efficacy published in 2012 in the Review of General Psychology (Vol 16(4) December 2012 364-338) which is the flagship journal published by the American Psychological Association. You can read more about it here: http://tapping4.us/research-feinstein. For more information on academic studies, visit the Resources section located at the back of the book.

Who can use EFT Tapping?

Everyone can benefit from tapping with EFT to ease your Migraine Headache signs. You may even aid others by performing the verbalization and tapping their symptoms. As with everything health-related, you must always consult a licensed physician prior to starting any new course, such as using EFT.

Is it safe for children to make use of EFT Tapping?

Anyone can benefit from tapping with EFT, even children to ease the Migraine Headache manifestations. It is possible to help those who are young to tap themselves by facilitating the verbalization and tapping on their behalf. But, like everything health-related, you must always consult a licensed medical professional before beginning an exercise program.

Is EFT safe to use? tapping for other purposes?

Within the normal limits of health-related issues it is recommended to consult with a medical professional who is qualified prior to starting any new program I'd say an overwhelming "yes!" I've personally employed EFT Tapping to deal with or ease symptoms from a myriad of ailments. I've helped people overcome the Fear of Flying, Fear of Heights as well as headaches, Headaches and much more. Gary Craig, the creator of EFT has always said, "Try it on everything!" And I'd be a resounding echo of that advice.

Which side should I tap which side should I tap on?

There is a consensus that it's not important what side you tap. I usually tap both sides and tap using two fingers, so I can cover more space as I tap. So, I don't need to be concerned about hitting the right area of my tapping and can focus on the problem at the moment instead.

How hard can I tap?

I usually tap using two fingers the same force as I use a computer keyboard when typing. I tap with two fingers to ensure I can cover more of the tapping area and I can concentrate on tapping as well as the Reminder Phrase instead of pondering if I'm actually getting the right tap location.

When should I begin tapping?

To treat Migraine Headaches I'd begin tapping right at the first indication that the headache is beginning. Most people be able to identify a series of emotions or sensations that can be an indication of the onset of a Migraine Headache. Personally, I'd begin to tap on these particular symptoms, as well as the "fear that I'm about to get a Migraine Headache."

Personally, I begin tapping whenever I see something I'd like to change. I'd suggest tapping while walking in order to take your regular Migraine Headache treatment or medication. There's a good chance that you've got only a couple of minutes between the moment you feel the Migraine getting worse and the time you begin your usual treatment plan to treat it, so you can try tapping (if you're willing to wait that long!)

How long should I tap?

The question is a bit difficult to be able to. At the beginning I'd suggest you tap until the symptoms go away. However, it is important to be accountable for your own health and your overall health and wellbeing. (As when it comes to anything that is health-related it is recommended to consult with a licensed medical professional prior to beginning any new exercise.) Therefore, a better option is to encourage you to spend at minimum in a couple of minutes of tapping prior to taking other steps to relieve. In the event that EFT Tapping is working for you and bringing you relief, I'd keep tapping and focus on possible ways I could come up with to tackle the issue, until I'd reached the goal of symptom relief. However If I was not noticing any noticeable change after a few minutes in tapping (maybe 3-4 times) then I'd consider other methods to relieve symptoms. It is a good idea to try EFT Tapping next time at the first indication of migraine symptoms.

When should I be tapping?

I would use EFT tapping anytime (and each) occasion that I noticed signs of symptoms of a Migraine Headache. If the symptoms disappeared but then returned and I would re-tap. The first person I taught on how to apply EFT tapping to treat a migraine was able to notice relief within a couple of minutes. But, she noticed that after a few hours, her symptoms started to get worse, so she tried EFT Tapping twice and had no migraine throughout the day. It's not a guarantee that is the case for you however, the important thing is she took exactly the "right thing" and tapped once more when her symptoms began to come back. She was rewarded for her efforts by being able to stop it from growing into something that was more severe. (As with any health-related issue it is recommended to consult with a certified medical professional prior to beginning any new exercise.)

How can I tell if it's working?

There are several ways to tell you are EFT Tapping is having the desired results. In the beginning, you're likely to observe the fact that your SUDS rating is decreasing which is a good indication that you're moving forward. You may also find yourself crying (or even vomiting!) while tapping. I've noticed it's a frequent occurrence for me, and is an indication that a "shift is happening." Thirdly, you might notice an exaggerated sigh or relaxation of your body. Fourth, you may experience changes in your perception or attitude regarding the subject. Things that were quite "big" for you simply don't seem to be a big deal to you now. Finally, you could just "notice a shift" and that's all you could describe it.

How should I proceed if I detect a shift?

The quick answer is to continue tapping your SUDS if it's not zero but! But, there are two main aspects to be considered which fall under an overall category called "how much have you shifted?"

If you've been completely shifted and can see that your SUDS for the issue is now zero, it's possible to think about resolving the issue. But, it's also an opportunity to look into it for a while to make sure that the issue is fixed, and that there aren't any other related issues that need to be worked to be addressed. If, for instance, I was working with someone about fears of spiders and they were at an absolute zero when they saw the spider then I would suggest asking the person to think about the experience to watch a spider move toward them, or moving away from them, or even walking towards them. Each of those might be related to one another and must be addressed simultaneously, while the primary focus remains the "fear of spiders." It's also an illustration to illustrate "taking a problem apart into its component pieces and then dealing with each one individually."

Then, if you've noticed a change but your SUDS isn't yet at zero (or at a minimum, very close) then I'd recommend tapping to pinpoint the problem. Also, I'd suggest including "...this additional information ..." as part of the Reminder and Setup Phrases. Sometimes, persistence is needed to truly "finish things off," however it's well worthwhile in my experience.

I noticed a shift in my initial impression but I'm still trapped...

If you've noticed a change initially however you are frustrated by your SUDS score not changing There are a few points to take into consideration.

The first thing you should check for is, have you moved to another part of the problem or a different problem entirely? Sometimes, I've seen myself doing this without being aware of it in the first place. Sometimes, it seems that the issue I'm tapping can be "so gone" that I do not even know the issue! These are the instances when it's somewhat confusing and illustrates more clearly the benefits in writing down the issue as well as the SUDS score prior to tapping.

If this isn't the case I'd suggest a second couple of times of tapping with the Setup Phrase and really saying it in a loud voice as you tap on the KC. Sometimes, we're stuck until there's a psychological shift to overcome the issue and, by doing so allows us to restart on the road to progress.

The next thing I'd look for is the scope of the problem. Sometimes, we attempt to tackle an issue that is larger and we get some results in the form of an SUDS reduction, only to hit a wall. It could be like EFT Tapping isn't working, however, you could be trying to tackle multiple aspects at the same time. I suggest to take a few minutes and determine if you can reduce the problem further into smaller components. For instance, I would not attempt to tackle the issue of "fear of flying" by tapping on "fear of flying" but instead, I'd like to break it down into components. According to my experience "fear of flying" may include sub-components such as anxiety about heights fear of the movement of the plane and not knowing what's about to occur, and not being in control (of the airplane or the environment) and perhaps even the smells of jet engine exhaust, which is often found in airports. There may be sub-components associated with memories of films TV shows, films as well as news articles. The sub-components can vary depending on the individual and what I'd suggest is to start with the you feel you feel is "most in your face" in terms of the SUDS intensity. When you feel that the SUDS intensity of this one decreases and disappears I'd then begin tap on the second powerful as well as the most "in your face" aspect that appears. It's probable that something like this could have multiple aspects, and each must be considered and tapped at individually as part of a larger sequence of tapping performed to help alleviate the general issue or symptoms.

Another way to approach this is to examine and determine if there's an explanation for why it's the case that it isn't "safe to get over the problem" which our subconscious is employing to protect the issue. A major part of the task of our subconscious is to "keep us safe" and it may react strongly to any thing it believes as an imminent threat to our security. These "threats" may be something that a child of 4 would consider is dangerous but it's not something that an adult would consider a threat. Therefore, they might seem strange at moments. For instance, if you begin to feel an Migraine Headache at the point that the time to visit your obstinate mother-in law is getting closer the subconscious might attempt to "keep you safe" by stopping you from being subjected to this scenario. This is a simple example I know, but it helps to illustrate the concept. The problem (or at the very least, the trigger) might not be in the place you think it should be, and it might not be apparent at all. Sometimes, these situations require some detective work to discover what the "real issue" to tap on.

Chapter 8: What Can I Do If I'm Unable To Notice An Alteration?

The first thing I'd like to think about is the problem or the definition in the first place. Is it too general or broad?

What I suggest is to look at the issue for a while and try to reduce the problem further into smaller components. For instance, I'd not tackle the issue of "fear of flying" by tapping on "fear of flying" but instead, I'd like to cut it up into its parts. It is also unlikely that I begin by tapping "this Migraine" but rather consider taking a moment to concentrate on the SUDS, the Character and the area. My experience is that a migraine may have sub-components as the "fear of flying" may contain a number of sub-components, such as anxiety about heights the movement of the aircraft as well as the sensation of turbulence, fear of being claustrophobic, not knowing what's likely to happen, and not being at the helm (of the plane or of the situation) and perhaps even the smells of jet engine exhaust which can be found often found in airports. There may be sub-components associated with the memories of films TV shows, movies or news reports.

If you are suffering from a migraine, or other physical condition I like to think of these sub-components from the perspective of character and location. As an example, in the description:

"A chronic and throbbing pain just behind and between the outside and the inside that lies above your left eye. It has an SUDS intensity rating of five. There is tension in your muscles that surround your scalp with a general SUDS of 3, however it's more intense to the left of your ear, with an SUDS of 4 in that region. Your vision may be somewhat "off" but full blown auras aren't yet happening so the 2."

The pain is described as having the "dull and throbbing" Character as well as the

Character that is associated with the head can be described as "muscle tension," and the Character that is associated with the symptom of vision is "slightly off." The location of the pain is "slightly behind and above the inside edge of your left eye," however there are two places that are that are associated with the tension in the muscles - "the scalp" in general as well as "on the scalp on the left side above your ear." The place of the issue with vision will be obvious to be your eyes. If you only have one eye, or a small portion or part of the vision appeared "slightly off," then it must be noted as the location.

The sub-components of these will differ between people and what I'd suggest is to start with the sensation that is "most in your face" in terms of SUDS strength. After it is apparent that SUDS intensity of this one diminishes and goes away I would then begin tapping on the next invigorating which is the "in your face," aspect that is evident. It's likely that something similar to this could have multiple aspects and each ought to be looked at and then tapped on separately in a collection of tapping.

The other thing I'd think about is to be determined. I'd try another time to two times with the Setup Phrase and really saying it in a loud voice, and then tapping the KC. Sometimes, we are stuck and there's a psychological shift in order to get over the issue . This can help us get back on the road to progress.

Another option is to examine the reason for why it's "not safe to get over the problem," which our subconscious might be trying to keep the problem. A major part of the task of our subconscious is to "keep us safe" and it can be quite adamant to anything it sees as threats to our security. These "threats" may be something which a four-year-old might think is dangerous but it's not for an adult. They may therefore seem strange at times.

If, for instance, you notice yourself gaining symptoms of Migraine Headache as the time to visit your mother-in-law who is a bit obnoxious is nearing Your subconscious might try to "keep you safe" by stopping you from being subjected to this circumstance. This is a simple example I know, but it illustrates the idea. The problem (or at the very least, the trigger) could not be exactly where you would expect it to be and may not be apparent at all. Sometimes, these issues require some investigation to identify what the "real issue" to tap on.

In the end, if any of the other options have resulted in a positive outcome I'd suggest minimum of three rounds of EFT tapping in full to "Even though I'm not making progress tapping on this issue, I deeply and completely love and accept myself, and I'm open to the possibility that whatever is blocking my progress will become obvious to me, so I can address it." I would repeat the Setup 3 times making sure to tap the KC and say"This" in a loud voice. Then , I'd go through at minimum three rounds of tapping making sure to tap every one of the standard EFT tapping points, and using the Reminder Phrase such as, "This Hidden Block." Then , I would stop to be still for a while and then look for an answer that arises in my mind. In most cases the process will result in some sort of insight that gets you moving forward. The insight could come after a while or perhaps in the coming days. When you tell your subconscious there is a chance of an answer coming to you in the future, you are inviting it to reveal the solution to you. Sometimes it takes some time because we're so busyand our minds are overflowing with information that our subconscious is having a hard time in finding the "open slot" to put the information so that it will be noticed by you! Give it some time and space, and you'll be amazed at what comes up!

How can I tell the moment it's "done" tapping?

On the surface it appears that the best answer is that you've "shifted completely" and you can see that your SUDS for the issue, has changed to an 0. It is tempting to believe that this issue is solved. But this is an opportunity to investigate the issue a bit more to ensure that it's fixed and there aren't any other related issues that need to be worked to be addressed.

For instance, if I was working with someone about the fear they have of spiders and they were at the point of having zero tolerance for seeing spiders I would suggest asking to think about the experience to watch a spider move towards, or away from them or walking towards them. Each of these might be connected and must be addressed in tandem, even though the main focus remains upon "fear of mice." It's also an illustration to illustrate "taking a problem apart into its component pieces and then dealing with each one individually."

Another thing I'd suggest is to find out whether you're able to "test it" to check whether the issue is gone. Begin by imagining in vivid detail the scenario. Try to exaggerate the your thoughts, sounds and sensations in the way you imagine it. If it doesn't create an emotion, then I'd suggest testing it in the real world , if you're able.

For instance, it's something to be able to be seated in your living space and "tap away" your fear of heights and believe that your fear is gone since you do not have a negative reaction when you imagine the scenario that caused the fear in the past. It's an entirely different matter to actually sit at the top of an observation deck in the Empire State Building looking over the railing's edge and taking in the panorama! Making sure you are safe on the spot is a good way to test what problem has been resolved. It is important to be accountable for your own safety and that of others as well, which is why you should "sneak up on" the items you're trying to test. If you do begin to receive a response while you're experimenting, in real life you should stop and perform tapping on the issue that happens to you before proceeding with any more testing or try to approach the situation more carefully. It's not necessary to "grit your teeth and push through it," since by using EFT Tapping you can release the issue more gently. It may require a few more times of tapping however, in the end it's well worth it to experience an emotional release from the issue!

Chapter 9: How Can I Be More Effective Using Eft Tapping?

First, I would suggest that we utilize EFT Tapping more often. It is common to experience minor irritations or emotional disturbances that pop up in the course of the course of the day. Although we often allow them pass over the following days or hours If we apply EFT Tapping for the emotional issue you can get rid of it quicker and also benefit by the effect of generalization which often occurs when tapping.

The thing that Gary Craig noticed over his long time of tapping as well as teaching tapping to others it is that there is an effect of generalization. For instance, if there are 100 trees within "the emotional upset forest of your past" it is likely that you will not have to deal with the entire 100 trees by using EFT tapping. It is possible that after addressing 10, 20, or 30 trees, the whole forest begins to fall apart. This is definitely among the "side benefits" of investing your time tapping. Tapping on these tiny things definitely helps get rid of the roots of a few of these trees, causing them to can fall much more quickly.

Another option is to pose the "Is there a previous similar circumstance to the one we are in now? In most cases, this question will trigger memories of a previous time when something similar took place which laid the foundation upon which the present issue is built. Similar to the real world in the event that you destroy the foundation and the remainder of the building will crumble. I will always look for and pursue these "earlier similar" incidents whenever I find these. The tapping on these issues can aid in bringing down further "trees in the forest" that are much more quickly.

Similar to this taking a step back and examining the tapping issue from a different angle, may give you insights, as well as additional tapping options, or routes towards success in removing the problems. Examining questions such as, "What would I lose, or gain?" or, "Who would be upset if I did or didn't achieve my goal?" will often yield interesting insights and tapable issues.

FAQ for Migraine Headaches

It's so painful that I'm afraid to tap my fingers Do you have a better way to do it?

There are a number of suggestions that I can offer in this instance.

The first step is to "touch and breathe" instead of tapping. Simply press the tapping area then breathe out and in for a time before moving to the next spot and repeating the same process. What this does is focus your focus on the area while you perform the breathing process and repeat your Reminder Phrase to yourself (or even imagining it if it's the only thing you have to do.)

It is possible to take this technique to the next step by tapping the spots and you imagine using the Reminder phrase loudly. This might not be as efficient as physically touching or tapping the spots, however in the event that it's all option, then it's the most effective thing you are able to accomplish. You may even find after taking the edge off of it and you're capable of physically tapping or touching those spots in the following step towards relief.

Another method you can do is watch the video of someone tapping, and then substituting the words "your issue" for the ones that are used on the screen. It is also helpful to imagine in your mind that you're tapping of your body to get the most effective result. If this helps to ease the pain for you, perhaps you can begin physically tapping while you focus on your problem using words.

Child's injuries are so severe that they're refusing to assist by tapping their backs.

What else can I do to help them through EFT?

(Please take note that even though I have focused my explanation on working with children however, this could be equally effective for adults.)

Yes, there are many ideas I could offer in this particular situation.

In the beginning, you can assist them with an alternative method called the "touch and breathe" technique instead of tapping. Simply press the tapping area and let them breathe in and out for a time before moving to the next tap point and repeating the process. This will focus their attention on the area as they go through an breathing pattern. You can repeat the Reminder Phrase to them to keep their attention on the problem. You can also tell them that they are able to mentally replace their own description of the problem (or the location, and character of the issue) while you do this. When it is done, and they have taken some of the tension off their shoulders, they might begin to repeat the descriptions and words loudly to you.

If they're not willing to even to touch them, attempt to take it step further by getting them to imagine tapping the spots while notifying the spot you are tapping by using your Reminder Phrase to them loudly. This may not be as efficient as physically touching or tapping the spots, however, in the event that it's what you can do at the moment, that's the best thing you can accomplish. You may even find once you've taken the edge off and you're able to go on towards physically tapping or touching on them to take the next step towards relief.

Another method you can do is have them observe you while you tap yourself to address their problem. While this might sound like a strange idea it could be the beginning of the journey towards relief. This is particularly true if you use your inner senses and go with your gut think you feel, or imagine what it might look like in the circumstance Tap using the words that pop into your mind to describe the situation. When it comes to kids and pain, be aware that it can be terrifying for children to be in this many pains and so confront that anxiety if you believe that it applies.

Other headache-related strategies and tips...

I'd like to share another couple of tricks I've come across. Check them out and see if they can benefit you.

The base of the tapping of the scull

A couple of years ago, a close friend of a friend was watching the first Migraine tapping video I created. The video was reported by her that the method didn't work for her as much as she had hoped until she added a second tapping area. She added tapping on the bony ridge located at the rear of the base of her skull. after she had added this she experienced a greater degree of relief.

In her message to me, she mentioned that as young and suffered from headaches her mother would tap and rub the area near the base of her skull. It's not clear to me if this is an actual "real tapping point," it's possible that there are meridians of energy acupuncture that pass through this area, or if it was just "her spot" as a result of her childhood.

The reason I have included this information is not only do i want to share all my "secrets" with you, however, I also want to remind you that everyone has many personal sources that we've not thought of. Take a look back at your own personal story and you could discover a gold nugget just like one that is waiting for you.

"Headache Point" on the hand

Many times I've heard about "the headache point" on the hand. It's located at the center of the skiny web that runs between your thumb and the side the hand. (In the near the area to the red triangular area in the image below.) This muscle is responsible for moving the thumb towards the hand's side. Although it is usually painful to do but some have reported substantial relief from headaches by rubbing and pinching the muscle inside that web.

I've heard it said that it can be more effective with either hand and you might be able to test applying pressure and massaging to the muscles across both hands. If one hand is more painful and tender over the others, it's thought to be the one to do the most.

It is often called "Trigger Point Therapy" in the massage industry. It's as bizarre as it sounds it is believed there exists an "headache Trigger Point" in the area. By applying pressure on this trigger spot (by pressing on it) it could eventually be released, and with it, relieve at the very least some of the headache pain.

The purpose is to exercise the muscle, then relax it by pressing this muscle with your thumb or the index finger of your other hand. You might want to consider massaging that entire (red triangle) region and the muscles beneath.

Tips, Tricks and Tips for using EFT tapping

In this section, I'm going to give you some of the tips techniques, tricks, and secrets that I employ when using EFT tapping. These are the simplest of things , and once you are aware about them, you'll be able to improve and get faster results from your EFT tapping.

Chapter 10: Floor-To-Ceiling Eye Roll Shortcut

In Gary Craig's initial training DVD's , he demonstrates an easy technique that most can prove very efficient in releasing the final part of the problem within a shorter time frame than the time it takes to perform an entire round of tapping. He typically applies it after the SUDS level was at the level of a one or two.

"floor-to-ceiling eye roll "floor-to-ceiling eye roll" is performed by keeping your head in a still position, beginning by directed down towards the floor, then slowly, in about 6 or so seconds then rolling them up until looking up at the ceiling (all while you keep your head steady) while continuously tapping at "the 9-gamut spot."

"The 9-gamut spot" is located on one side of the hand between the knuckles. This in the area where the "ring finger" and "baby finger" meet. There is kind of a groove there that you tap on continuously while doing the floor-to-ceiling-eye-roll.

The next time you see your SUDS intensity is lower than either a 1 or 2 test it and check out what you think. Sometimes, it is effective with only one session; at other times, it requires several attempts. If the floor-to-ceiling-eye-roll is not resolving the issue and bringing the SUDS to a zero, then go ahead and do a regular round of EFT Tapping instead.

In addition to this publication, I made two videos to show the Floor-to-Ceiling Eye Roll in a more clear way than could be accomplished using just words and photos. You can see the first Floor-To-Ceiling Eye Roll video here: http://tapping4.us/eyeroll. The second Floor-To-Ceiling Eye Roll video is a more close-up shot where you can see my eye position more clearly, and it can be found here: http://tapping4.us/eyeroll2. There is a complete video list and other web-based content within the Resource section.

Finger Tapping Points

When Gary first developed EFT the company also included five additional tapping points for the hand. but they aren't used much in the present. But, they're useful to be aware of in particular as alternatives to tapping points. Alongside the 9-Gamut point mentioned above There are tapping points on the index finger, thumb middle finger, the index finger and the little finger. (The finger's meridian in the finger that is the ring is located at a different spot in the human body.)

It is possible to tap on these points as an addition to or as a substitute for tapping on other points. This can be especially useful for those who suffer from Migraine Headache signs and don't want to tap your head or face. Instead, try tapping with finger points. The process is similar tapping, focusing on the issue , and then repeating the Reminder Phrase, just like the normal EFT tapping technique that is described throughout the book.

Finger tapping, or massaging or rubbing your finger pointscan be employed in public in order to appear more discreet or cover up the tapping you're doing. Just focus on the problem, or the person, or the location in case of physical discomfort, and "think out loud" the Reminder Phrase while you're rubbing or tapping your fingers.

To add more information to this book, I've created an instructional video that shows the locations of tapping on the fingers more clearly than could be accomplished with photos and words by themselves. You can see the finger tapping locations video here: http://tapping4.us/hand. You can access a comprehensive list of videos as well as other web content under the section Resources.

Mental Tapping

It's easy to do at any time, from anywhere, without anyone noticing the exact method you're using. If tapping with your hands seems "not possible" or would cause disruption, you can imagine vividly doing tapping in the place. If you're using this technique to treat migraine symptoms, make certain to concentrate on the person, the place, and the character when you are mentally tapping. The trick is to imagine tapping each point as vividly as you can. Closing your eyes can help increase your concentration and eliminate distractions as you tap on each one. It is common to see results within minutes by mental tapping. It can be more difficult than tapping however, it can be highly efficient.

The use of mental tapping could also be an escape from the shame that comes with tapping out in the public. If you're finding that your tapping with your mind isn't going in the way you'd like it to, an alternative is to remove yourself from the situation and tapping somewhere on your own. Bathrooms are an ideal "hiding place" for tapping.

The public taps are not embarrassing.

A few additional words on how to tap "in public" without feeling embarrassed? If that question pops up my first reaction will always be: Tap on "feeling embarrassed about tapping in public!" Once everyone has gotten through that "Yeah, DUH!" moment, I continue to suggest that instead of tapping the points, you can imagine tapping the same points we've just have discussed.

A side note: In the book Entangled Minds by Dean Radin Doctoral student Dean Radin. He provides information about research that shows the brain can't distinguish between actual and vividly imagined events. Entangled Minds is available through Amazon.com: http://tapping4.us/eminds. You can tap with your mind while vividly picturing your fingers tapping at every point, and you will be able to cause the issue reduced the likelihood of it being solved! Stay focused and persist in it.

Free Online Resources

There are plenty of tapping resources to be found on the internet. There are even a lot of tapping videos available on YouTube. Due to the fact that EFT is so simple to master, a lot of people want to share their knowledge with their friends. However, there are times when it is the case that this "second-hand EFT" is incorrect or may be incorrect. Therefore you should be careful when choosing which information to focus on.

There are plenty of script ideas for tapping along with Setup Phrase examples in the article.

The most important thing to remember will be that you are getting an extensive archive that contains hundreds of pages of excellent material gathered by Gary as cases studies and examples of using EFT in real-life situations. You can utilize cases studies in order to discover other phrases to tap, as well as see how others have tackled their own issues using EFT tapping.

Tapping Journal

Utilize a simple $0.99 journal to track your migraine symptoms' Character, Location and SUDS. This is not just helpful for you at the beginning, when you're just beginning to learn about EFT tapping for Migraine symptoms However, by taking additional notes about what you did during the daily routine (what did you consume, your stress levels, changes in weather and so on.) there may be several common themes that you can tackle using EFT tapping or other methods (like cutting it out of the diet.)

Once you begin tapping with EFT Tapping to address issues that go beyond migraine symptoms Not only can you make use of your journal for tapping to record topics for the future sessions of tapping, but also keeping track of your progress will motivate you to continue tapping, and will remind you of the improvements you've achieved. If you come across subjects that you want to tap, note them down. You can use it while you're actively tapping but you can also record points to consider later when you're not able to tap them at the moment. It can be used to create "areas for exploration" when you're still not prepared to "dig in" to them however you do not want to lose them in the future.

Chapter 11: Speak The Truth Being Politically Incorrect In Your Words

You must be "Politically Incorrect" with your words to get better results in a shorter time! This is particularly true when you're focusing on reducing the stress you feel with a focus on Migraine symptoms prevention. There are numerous occasions in our lives when we are afraid to speak, and what we truly would like to say in order to appear politically correct or to be socially acceptable in the particular situation. When you're tapping particularly by yourself, be honest about your true feelings while you tap! Let your voice be heard! Find your Inner Sailor and go ahead and scream like a lunatic! You may have never been safe to express fully the emotions you felt. Now is the right time to connect with your feelings to let go! There's no reason for you to appear "Politically Correct" when tapping particularly if you're with yourself.

If, for instance, you're getting into more shape, do not spend your time focusing on "I don't like to exercise" instead of stating that you think "Exercise is a pain in the ass!" Tap instead! This is your truth in the end!

You're likely to see more results if you are able to really feel the feelings you feel! You will be able to be aware of the issue whenever you're "venting about it." It is likely that you begin "heated" and end up looking a bit ridiculous! Particularly when you are talking about it in what I refer to as"a "tap-and-bitch session." This change from being heated to a bit silly is a great thing since it means that things change!

A brief story to share here. A while ago, I was really, (did I mention REALLY really) angry and upset with myself over an ongoing issue. It was a blaze of anger all morning long until I entered my shower I was unable to take it anymore, and I took on my own venom, as I was tapping. It was an "tap-and-bitch session" in the shower. I was shocked by how quickly SUDS level and view changed. I don't think I've ever acknowledged to myself the level of frustration and anger I felt in my own mind about this subject. But I sure did on that day. Since I was completely at peace, it was obvious the fact that I had been "tuned into the issue" and within a matter of minutes, there was a massive decrease in the intensity of my anger and frustration. I don't think I reached the 4th or 3rd moment, where I did several taps to the KC and expressing my discontent, the level of frustration changed between "about a 15" down to around a 7 and then dropped quickly and then drop further. At the end of the day I had to confess to myself that, even though I was not happy with the manner in which things were unfolding however, I was doing my best did ... at the moment.

This is something we can often forget We're doing our best at the moment even though it might appear to be. To prove that is the question: when was the last time you decided to make a poor job on something that you are passionate about or want to see results from? I'm betting that you perform your absolute "best" that you can currently every day (even when it might not appear like it to someone else.)

If you want to change your reaction towards outside (and internally) stressors, you might consider making a final run of EFT tapping, beginning with tapping the KC as you say "Even though I may not like what's going on, I deeply and completely love and accept myself, and I acknowledge that we really are doing the best we can, even though it may not look like it!" Tap through several rounds, in a series of Reminder Phrases "doing the best we can" and "even though it may not look like it" while you tap. What I've noticed personally is that this is a perfect finish to this type of tapping and also decreases my stress level by further.

Tap-And-Bitch

It's a quick and easy method of releasing anger angry, irritated, or frustrated whenever it occurs. It's a great method to decrease stress levels and possibly prevent Migraine-related symptoms from surfacing. If "life gets crappy" and you've got something that you need to "bitch about," simply "tell the story" of the things you're angry about while tapping the entire of the time! Continue to tap through all pointsrepeatedly time till you "take the emotional charge off it" and it's less of a sour note. Better yet, continue tapping until you're completely neutral regarding the issue. A state of being "neutral" may show up as being bored by the subject or story.

Parents - This is great with children, and even their small "boo-boo" injuries! Let them tell the incident while tapping their feet. "Tap-and-tell" is the kid suitable variant that is similar to "Tap-and-bitch."

I would like to share with you a story I experienced myself that has convinced me to adopt this way of thinking. Jennifer's son was just 5 years old when he fell off the tree he was on. After having checked the tree to make sure that the only injury was the pride of his father, we inquired of the boy what happened. Through his tears and, of course, using his amazing 5-year-old brain and reasoning, he told us how he blamed his fall from the tree to his brother who was watching him through of the windows at that moment. As he explained the situation, Jen started tapping on his EFT points as he recounted the story. She encouraged him to retell the story many times while tapping him. After perhaps the third or fourth retelling He said he was dissatisfied and asked to return to climb up the tree once more! The most amazing thing about this story was that the fact that there was absolutely no hesitation for him about whether or not to "get back on the horse that threw him" so to speak, as so many children do after traumatizing falls such as the one he experienced. Even to this day he isn't afraid about climbing up trees! To me, this is an additional proof point to the effectiveness of tapping into the present moment to eliminate any trauma that is stuck and could "leave a mark" for the duration in your lifetime.

Since I'm convinced that this is a potent method that can be utilized to ease your stress quickly, I developed a website that is focused on this technique. You can find it at http://www.TapAndBitch.com and you when you enter your name and email address in the box in the upper right-hand corner of the site, you will be sent access to a free, 23-minute video that I created called The EFT Quick Start Video Learning System. I highly recommend you take a look. (Not to be a crude or offensive however "TapAndComplain.com" simply doesn't have the same impact, and isn't quite as memorable.)

Borrowing Benefits

It is possible to "get your tapping work done" by focusing at someone else tapping their problem. "Borrowing the Benefits" is accomplished by tapping alongside others who are addressing the concern. It might sound strange at first, but Gary Craig has witnessed how efficient it is numerous times, and has even demonstrated the technique through one of his instructional videos.

The first step is to find a video of someone tapping their problem. You can use the

Migraine tapping videos, or any other tapping videos I have referenced within this guide. You can even look on YouTube to find the EFT Tapping video that is like the issue you're trying to address.

Choose a symptom or issue that's bothering you and then give the issue an SUDS rating. You can also take note of the SUDS character, symptom and location in the case of an issue with a physical aspect. It may not be related to the issue recorded. Begin by tapping as you record with your attention on the issue and using their phrases. After you have completed the tap-along, review your problem and it is very likely that the issue has moved a bit, and might be down by some SUDS points as well.

This method is a sure thing. you can actually tap on something totally not related to the issue you're trying to address but still achieve amazing results! If you put your issue in your the forefront before you tap along with others the subconscious mind can "apply" the tapping to the issue you chose to focus on prior to tapping. Mindfulness is a wonderful thing!

It is also possible to use this method to assist others, like an infant, by taking them through the process with you. You might possibly be the person who is doing the tapping, and they could follow the process. Before starting it, you could pose a question similar to "If you had a magic wand that could make this tapping apply to anything, what would it be?" This would help keep the child's attention on the issue , even if they aren't willing to reveal the reason! Then, ask the child if they would like to have you tap along with you and then start tapping "your issue" even if you need to create it!

It's possible that you won't get results as quickly as you tackled the issue head-on however it's a start! If you can earn some SUDS points while chatting with another person, and you don't need to "confront your issues," go for this opportunity!

Chapter 12: What Is Eft?

EFT can be described as it's the Emotional Freedom Technique, also known as tapping. It's akin to psychological acupressure. an extremely unique technique to assist with a myriad of physical and emotional problems.

When we go through an "trauma" in our lives It could be minor, or have an impact that can change your life. Traumas could be as small such as witnessing your parents fight as an infant, or that has a greater impact, like witnessing a violent incident. If trauma is experienced and an emotion is disturbed, it is like an electric jolt to the system. The emotion that caused the trauma will become part of our bodies, and is weaved in the fabric of lives.

Some people describe trauma as a state of mind or emotion that becomes stuck within our nervous system and within our minds, leaving an impression left on our brains as a stamp leaves an impression of a memory. This makes sense since there are many memories from our past that come up in our minds when we see ourselves in certain circumstances.

A prime example is Post Traumatic Stress Disorder (PTSD). For instance, a lot of soldiers come back from battle and are able to re-enter the world, hoping to return to the way their lives were like prior to their deployment. But, they've endured trauma that a lot of us won't be able to comprehend. The study in which they compared the conventional therapy offered to military personnel, and the treatment that was offered to civilians along with EFT. It was found that those who employed EFT together with their regular therapy helped people suffering from PTSD recover much more quickly. There are also individuals who have traveled to Rwanda to assist children who witnessed their parents be killed. They now must assist the younger ones by playing the parental role as a child. It is easy to imagine how stressful it would be to have difficult time not only being a child who is hurting and also having to take on additional obligations. This group has put in place therapy programs for children, and they continue to make significant progress towards not just being able to manage their current circumstances and be hopeful about their future.

When we perform the tapping at acupressure points', we let go of the old stuck or

"stuck" emotions, and we give ourselves the chance to compose a new message. There are many advantages to EFT that can help with emotional issues and physically, however many have experienced positive effects of EFT on physical problems as well!

The Benefits of EFT

EFT can provide many healing benefits such as:

Non-evasive.

Simple and straightforward, it's impossible to make the job "wrong".

Learn the tricks in a brief time.

It is possible to do this at anytime, anywhere and on any subject.

It's a powerful tool that can produce lasting impact.

The effects that come with it are almost always positive.

EFT isn't a cure it or "cure" things, but it can help ease anxiety that can be caused by

issues, whether they are an issue with memory or stress-related. This is evident in the medication taken by people, the medications don't always cure problems, but it can help ease symptoms. EFT helps reduce stress and anxiety and can at times identify at the source of your issue. It may take some time however if you're perseverant and persistent, you'll probably see the improvements you're looking for.

History

The Dr. Roger Callahan in California Psychotherapist Dr. Roger Callahan in California has been teaching for more than 30 years ago the practice of Thought Field Technique (TFT). He was able to work with the thoughts of patients and integrated Acupuncture Points. The doctor. Callahan devoted much of his time learning and helping people suffering from various anxiety, fears and trauma, stress and many more.

Doctor. Callahan had a patient, Mary, who was terrified to death of water. This meant taking baths and going outside in the stormy weather. After seeking assistance in different ways, she was able to overcome her fear of the water by using this technique together with the doctor. Callahan. Following his session with Mary she was led to a swimming pool in is in the same location, and she did not show any signs of anxiety! This discovery inspired to Dr. Callahan to research more and eventually discover and develop patterns by tapping on Acupressure points. Then, he started teaching this method in the 80's.

Gary Craig, who was one of Gary Craig, who was one of Dr. Callahan's pupils in the 1990's, embraced the concept and streamlined it into what is now known as EFT. Gary is a key player in introducing this technique into the world via his workshops, web site and many other.

EFT is currently used by many people who use various variations. I am of the opinion that there is no "right" way to use EFT or "tapping". There are those who be skeptical but the fact that I've employed this with children and have had great outcomes proves to me that this technique isn't required to be performed precisely. This is why you'll be able to relax knowing that you don't need to be concerned over "doing it wrong". We'll go over different ways of tapping later within the text.

How It Works

Our bodies are energy which is fuelled by food and also an energy system driven by electrical impulses which flow through our bodies. When our body's system is not in balance and we're off balance, it's a sign that we're out of. Feeling "off balance" can show manifest in a variety of manners, emotionally as well as physically.

As a car requires to be tuned up and we also require the same treatment to maintain our balance. If our bodies and our emotional wellbeing aren't aligned well, they could cause imbalance.

appear in many types, such as fears and phobias, stress, depression, anger and anxiety. They can manifest in different forms such as guilt, stress and many more.

It is also possible to experience physical discomfort that manifests as a result of tension, which can manifest as tension, headaches, pain or illness, as well as all associated emotions. EFT can help with some of these emotional as well as physical problems.

We don't declare we can prove that EFT "cures" people, but it does relieve sufferers of their symptoms.

This approach has proved to be an invaluable resource for people fighting cancer. With cancer, there are many who struggle with not just the painful adverse effects of treatment but also the emotional side of hurt, anger and a myriad of negative emotions. Being in a positive mood can be very beneficial when trying to heal from an unpleasant treatment. More than 90% of those who make use of EFT who undergo treatment experience a positive outcome.

I've tried these techniques to help myself. At times, I suffer from back and neck pain , and EFT provides me with relief. In the past, I've utilized this method whenever I'm angry. Taps help me increase my patience and keep me in a calm state. It's so simple and user-friendly that I've used it when I was at the stoplight!

There's plenty to be learned about the procedure and the way it came about however, it can remain simple and straightforward when you are looking to do things right away to result in positive and lasting results.

Chapter 13: Tapping Basics

The Pressure Points

The order of points:

1. Karate Chop Point Karate Chop Point (Set-up the Statement) Tap the palm's soft side.

2. Eyebrow - You can tap it on both sides, in the the bridge of the nose

3. Eye Side - On bone

4. Under the eye - on bone

5. Under the Nose

6. Chin - Just below the lip

7. Collarbone - On the collarbone's knobs (bow the tie region)

8. Under the Arm Four inches below arm

9. top of head - crown of the head

Set-Up Statements and Sequence

1. The Set-Up Statement while tapping on the karate chop point, repeat the following statement three times. It is possible to modify the phrase to fit your style and requirements.

"Even though I have this (insert problem/issue), I accept myself."

2. The sequence: Tap six to eight times on each of the points and remain focused on the issue. The problem can be stated either within your head.

3. Examine Your emotions: Take a deep breathe and assess your mood on the scale 1-10. What did you think of your rating changing? Repeat the procedure to see if the intensity is still there or if additional concerns come to mind. It is possible that while you press on one subject an issue or memory could occur.

Prepare to continue through the process until all the aspects of the issue are addressed.

Borrowing Benefits

If you're working with a person one-on-one or in a group using EFT You can avail what's known as "Borrowing Benefits". I observed this happen while teaching classes in the past. If the whole room was focusing on the same subject, it might not be something who everyone could identify with. However, what's remarkable is that people can be relieved when working together. What is the reason? It could be that they weren't aware that the issue they had to deal with this problem or some similar one however they felt an increase in their energy. It could also be because they keep their personal issues at the forefront of their mind when tapping with others and are working on matters that aren't connected to the issues being discussed in the group. In any case, they gain.

Reviewing The Steps in Tapping

Define the fear, memory, or emotion you would like to address.

Determine the actual motivation of the emotion or fear. Look back to the most recent time that you were experiencing the problem or stress over the issue.

Create a target statement that will resolve the fear or memory by using your own words, along with any reactions you feel. What are your physical reactions when you think about this particular issue?

Determine the severity of the fear, memory or issue on the scale of 0-10.

Tap the points to get rid of the memory/issue/fear.

Repeat as often as you need to.

Putting It Into Practice

It is likely that you bought this book due to the fact that you are extremely frustrated with your organization or inability to organize. Perhaps you've been trying to organize numerous times in the past. You might have hired someone to come to your house, such as a professional organizers and with their help you managed to organize your home. After a few months or even years. It returned to the point it was before it was changed.

I've always believed that there's so much more to our possessions than just the material. There are many emotions that can be connected to our belongings. However, with clutter are other problems that are associated with being organized. They include feeling overwhelmed, procrastinating and having difficulty making decisions, and much more.

The pain that we've experienced in our lives may be related to the way we live in the present. I often hear about people who were in the depression and hold on to the most they could. It's understandable because they went through a period when they weren't able to get what they wanted and didn't want to experience that same pain. However, they're only causing themselves more discomfort by clinging to items and living in the fear.

When we put EFT in practice, we won't just focus on organizing-related issues as well as tackle physical and emotional concerns. Be aware that the words may be modified to suit your preferences and, even in the event that you do not alter the language, you'll get the benefits of borrowing.

Storytelling

Don't worry about expressing your thoughts "correctly". When you are going through every EFT session, I'd like you to reflect on the way you tell your story, and the way you're communicating what's within your mind and in your heart as if you were telling your own story.

Your story is telling about your origins as well as how you are feeling right now, and how you would like to experience in the coming years. When you consider the EFT rounds that way, it will be easy for you to create your own personal words when you are at ease doing it.

You can share your story while you tap on each of the points. I've had this experience myself. I've noticed that when I am tapping and speaking about the issue or stress I'm experiencing it is possible to find solutions. This is something that amazes me. However, it isn't right. It's similar to praying. I'm focused and asking to be clear and directing. When I talk about gratitude and acceptance during my tapping sessions even if I don't notice it at the time it will bring me peace.

If you're not sure what you can pray for or who to ask you, or if you're in a state of confusion, telling your story is the best way to gain clarity and perhaps some suggestions for moving forward.

Before we start I'd like you to make an inventory of the memories that have a negative impact on your. Spend 30 minutes or so to write down a complete list of all the memories you'd like to transform from a negative experience to positive ones. Focus on organization issuesand then create an additional list of any additional memories that you wish to tackle. I recommend keeping journals or notebooks. Writing down your list of dates and results will help you remember how far you've made when you revisit and look through your old entries.

Chapter 14: Areas Of Organization

Clutter

Clutter can be more than just a pile of papers or a messy closet. Clutter could be a sign of being uneasy and uncertain. It could be a sign of wanting to keep yourself safe from strangers entering your home or your space. It could also represent the need to avoid the potential dangers that lie right in front of you and can scare you. What do your clutter says about you and your circumstances?

It's not just about your personal space as well as your schedule. It can as well your physical and emotional wellbeing.

It can create a line around them that prevents them from progressing. Even though they might say that they are unhappy with the mess, they will continue to make use of it as a reason to avoid other activities.

Write down questions you have asked yourself/jot in notebook:

What do you think your clutter has prevented the you from doing?

What are you going to do with your mess or disorder to justify your clutter or disorganization?

If you were well-organized What could you achieve?

Examples include:

What would happen if there was the space to start my business, and it could make it

What is the outcome when I ate healthy and was taking care of myself what could I expect from me?

PRACTICE

Tapping on Feeling Embarrassed About Clutter

Karate Chop:

1. While I'm embarrassed by my clutter,

I accept myself as I am.

2. Although I'm sure I must hide it from guests,

I accept who I am in all honesty.

3. Even though I'm shamed and ashamed about my mess,

I accept who I am in all honesty.

Eyebrows: I'm embarrassed of my brows.

The other side of the eye Eye side: I don't wish to host guests.

In the corner: I do not think of what I should do.

In the dark The only thing I know is I'm hiding it.

Chin: As with me, I have many other qualities about myself.

Collarbone The reason I'm embarrassed by my junk.

The arm that is under the table: I'm afraid I'm embarrassed of myself.

Head to the top: I'd like I want to release.

Eyebrows: I'd like to make a fresh start.

Eye side Eye side: Let me go of guilt over the clutter that I have accumulated.

Eyes I'm exhausted of being embarrassed.

The truth is that it may take some time to bring the mess to a manageable level, but now I'm on the verge of being ready.

Chin Then I'm sick of being a victim of excuses and hiding my lifestyle.

Collarbone The Collarbone are going to change, and I'll be released.

Under the arm The first step of admitting that I'm guilty.

The top of my head: I'll continue to work towards creating an environment that is relaxing and clutter-free.

Take a nice deep breath.

Tapping on Letting Go

Karate Chop:

1. While I'm having a difficult time getting rid of my belongings,

I am okay with myself.

2. Even though I was pressured to give up things before I was fully prepared,

I'm okay with me.

3. Although it is difficult for me to release my old habits,

I'm ok with what I feel now.

Eyebrow: What if require my items later on?

Eye side The other side of the eye: I'm wasting my time even if I'm throwing them away!

Eyes: I would like to keep my things.

In the nick of time: I don't think about when I might require them.

Chin If I save everything and did not use them.

Collarbone It's it's a waste of space grasp everything.

The arm is under the table: What is the case if I really need it and need to purchase another one?

Top of the head It's an item and I'm not going to throw it away. I'd be wasteful of money.

Eyebrow: I'm sure I might be able to donate the brow to someone else who would benefit from it.

Eye side Side of the eye: I can offer a small amount at one time.

Eyes: If I took it just a tiny amount at a time, it wouldn't be like it was so overwhelming.

At a price that isn't the most annoying thing is that I could need to purchase another.

Chin: I'm the only one with all my memories, and no one is able to take them away.

Collarbone Think of the space I'll gain and less to rummage through.

The arm is under my back: take a small amount at a time, which is doable.

Head to the top: It's simply stuff and I'll never forget my memories. I'm ready to feel liberated.

Take a deep breath.

Tapping on Clutter Habits

Karate Chop:

1. Although I do have this habit of not throwing objects away I am ok with my own shortcomings.

2. Although I do have a problem with clutter, I'm accepting myself regardless.

3. Although I'm not sure what I can do to improve I'm determined to improve myself and accept myself for who I am.

Eyebrows: I don't need to look perfect.

Eye side Eye side: I'm just trying to be efficient and consistent.

Eyes I'm not fond of the mess around me.

The naivete The nose: This is a bad habit I have.

Chin: I'm confused about how to stay organized or utilize my time effectively.

Collarbone: I'm trying to change my perception of me.

In the Arm There's still time to develop these ways of life.

The top of my head Top of the head: My life can be completely different with the introduction of new ways of living.

Eyebrow: I'm ready alter the way I live my life.

The other eye Side of the eye: I am thrilled to implement these changes.

Under the eyes I'm ready to make a change.

The truth is that I'm eager to try all my new routines.

Chin The way I live my life will gradually change to the better and I will eventually be clear.

Collarbone It is my goal to stop the habit of being chaotic.

The arm is now in my hand The goal is to be less anxious and less stressed.

Heads up: I'm looking forward to creating new habits that are right for me! I'll come up with a fresh method to be inspired by my surroundings and the way I live my life.

Take a nice deep breath.

Tapping on Where to Start

Karate Chop:

1. While I'm overwhelmed and I'm not sure where to begin, I'm here for everyone of me.

2. Despite the fact that there's so much to do that I am overwhelmed I'm accepting my situation regardless.

3. While I'm not sure where to begin and find myself feeling defeated but I'm accepting the whole me.

Eyebrow: I'm overwhelmed and depressed I'm overwhelmed and don't want to take on anything.

Eye side The eye has so much to take in, including all my piles.

Under the eyes: It's difficult to figure out where to start.

Then, do I do it on my own , or do I solicit assistance?

Chin What would happen if I only did one thing, or one stack?

Collarbone The Collarbone through just one stack.

The arm is under my body: could do one pile and then stop for breaks.

The top of my head I could return and complete an additional pile in the future.

Eyebrows: It makes me feel like I'm in a panic if I do it wrong.

The side of the eye When I throw away some thing I wanted, I would be able to find another.

Under the eyes: I like it when I see less piles.

The nose I'll feel so much better once I start!

Chin The simple act of starting can boost my confidence and help me feel better.

Collarbone: I'm going to start with one pile at one time.

Chapter 15: Procrastination

Procrastination does not cause the problem. It is a symptom of the issue. If you can identify the reasons behind why you delay the opportunities in front of you, you'll be able to move ahead. In order to solve the issues that you might have concerning procrastination, I would suggest that you create an outline of the items and goals that you've put off. No matter how you've put off it off, simply record it. Did you have something you have given up on? Note it down. It's a great release to write everything down on newspaper or in your notebook.

Write down a question you want to ask yourself or write in your notebook:

What will happen if this project was completed?

What are the negatives to carrying out this task and getting it done?

It's fear of failure or anxiety about success.

Examples:

I could be criticized or judged by people around me.

People can be jealous, or angry (family friends, spouse.)

I may become more prosperous, but too busy, or will not visit my family.

I'm not sure what I'd be if I shed weight, found a job, and earned my degree.

I don't like committing.

I feel trapped.

PRACTICE

Tapping on Procrastination

Karate Chop:

1. Although I am aware that I must take a decision, I'd rather sit and wait,

I accept myself as I am.

2. Even though I'm feeling stuck and stuck and I can't get my feet moving,

I accept who I am in all honesty.

3. While I'd prefer to delay things instead of moving forward,

I am the person I am at this moment.

Eyebrows: I'm angry with myself.

Eye side Side of the eye: It's clear what I have to accomplish, however I'm not sure how to perform it.

Under the eyes How do I plan to progress and achieve my goals?

In the face I'm overwhelmed by the issue, which leads to me avoiding it through procrastination.

Chin Chin: It's more easy to ignore and avoid the things that need to be taken care of but I really would like it to be solved.

Collarbone: I am sure I could complete these tasks however I chose not to.

The arm is under the table: I'm not content with my decision to not to participate in projects, because this choice doesn't serve me.

Top of the head I'm looking to decide how I will take a step forward.

Eyebrows: I must be free of the habit of procrastinating.

The side of the eye The eye is preventing me from being my best.

In the blink of an eye: I can accomplish lots of things by defeating procrastination.

In the nick of time: I don't need to do this in a perfect way.

Chin: I'm pretty sure that's the reason why I'm staying clear of this. I'm scared of causing a mess.

Collarbone: I'm aware that it's necessary to do it even if I make mistakes.

The arm is under the arm I'll feel much better after this is finished.

The top of your head It'll be so liberating to be done!

Take a nice deep breath.

Tapping on Avoidance

Karate Chop:

1. While I may avoid certain situations or tasks I am incredibly happy with the person I am in all of them.

2. Although I do not like things that have to be accomplished, I sincerely and completely accept myself as I am.

3. While I am always waiting to see if the things happen by themselves, I am content with what I am at this moment.

Eyebrows: I'm angry with myself.

The side of the eye Side of the eye: I'm not sure why I decided to stay clear of situations.

Under the eyes I hope in my heart that it will vanish.

In the nick of time: I don't need to handle it, or that someone else will.

Chin: Except no one else does.

Collarbone Perhaps if I had the courage I had to accomplish the job, it would be accomplished.

In the arms: Perhaps If I had the certainty in the knowledge that I made the right choice then the right choice was made.

Top of the head I'm trying to decide how I will take a step forward.

Eyebrow When I stop looking at my eyebrows, I can actually finish a task that I don't want to do.

Eye side Side of the eye: Even though I don't enjoy working on certain projects I might get help or understand the things I need to accomplish.

Eyes: I'm sure avoidance isn't the solution.

In the midst Imagine what I could accomplish if I simply did what I had to accomplish.

Chin The issue isn't easy to avoid or ignore since it's always in my back mind.

Collarbone The Collarbone assistance and support.

Under the arm: I'll feel so happy knowing that I can finally complete what is needed to be completed.

The top of my head is that I believe this opens up new possibilities for me since I was forced to confront what I was not prepared for. I'm very excited about that.

Take a nice deep breath.

Overwhelm

The feeling of overwhelming is the sensation that there is "too much". It is possible to feel overwhelmed by the noise or lack of space too many things to do or too many choices. This is something that is too much for a person.

What do you think your life would look like if you weren't overwhelmed often? Everyone feels overwhelmed from time to time. If, however, you experience it regularly, it's time to take a step back and consider what it's doing to your. Feeling overwhelmed may feel like feeling anxious. It's not a pleasant feeling. If you learn to use this sensation as a way to gauge your state and recognize when it's time to review the cause that's contributing to feeling overwhelmed.

In addition to identifying situations in which you are overloaded, employ tapping to help you find your center to get yourself out of the feeling that you are not in control. This is exactly what it is, feeling like you are out of control.